Therapists and Parents Praise *Pilates For Parenting*

Pilates for Parenting—what a brilliant concept! We are all very aware of how important it is for us to exercise to keep our bodies fit and healthy. We join gyms, take classes, develop daily disciplines all in an effort to better care for ourselves. So why not take the same approach to our most important role, parenting.

As this powerful little book points out, from the moment your child enters the world you *are* the most important person in your child's life. *Pilates for Parenting* teaches simple yet powerful exercises that will help you strengthen your parental core. Implementing the exercises will help you develop daily disciplines to become more aware and mindful of your role as a parent. **Pilates for Parenting by Holli Kenley is a must have resource for all parents and guardians.**

Jed Doherty, Executive Producer and Host of
Reading With Your Kids Podcast www.readingwithyourkids.com

Pilates For Parenting is a perfect guide to help parents foster better relationships with their children. I particularly like Holli's explanation about 'showing-up' for our children. For example, in the digital age in which we live, we are often too distracted by our smartphones, social media sites, and television screens. We model this behavior for our children and our children wind up following the same path. As a result we become more and more disconnected from the ones we love. **Pilates For Parenting just might be the best method for reconnecting with your children and developing stronger relationships.**

Thomas Kersting, MA, LPC
Author, *Disconnected: How to Reconnect Our Digitally Distracted Kids*

I wish I had read this book when my (now adult) daughter was younger. Only now do I better understand her need for attention and affirmation when we were dealing with other family matters. *Pilates For Parenting* guides the reader through all types of family dynamics, shedding light on common, current, and perplexing issues. Holli combines solid information with personal questions, for the reader to ponder and put into practice. **The text, workouts, activities and guiding exercises in *Pilates for Parenting* will equip readers with their own personalized, practical, effective game-plan as they navigate the ups and downs of becoming nurturing, protective and wise parents.** The one powerful quote I'll always remember, gives me hope, and pertains to future growth: "It's never too late for a redo. NEVER!"

Judy Herzanek, Changing Lives Foundation
Co-author, *Why Don't They Just Quit? Hope for families struggling with addiction*

One of the most challenging things I encounter as a play therapist is how to encourage parents to take a hard look at themselves and at the same time strengthen their bond with their children. This book gives caregivers permission to take the time to do just that.

Holli Kenley's new book *Pilates for Parenting* hits the nail on the head when it comes to what questions we can ask ourselves to make sure our children know they matter to us and that we are listening to what they have to say to us. This is an invaluable resource for parents and caregivers to improve their relationships with their children, focus on what they believe is best for their children, and support their children in growing into confident adults.

This is not your normal "how to" parenting book. *Pilates For Parenting* **helps us as caregivers get to the heart of our parenting, take time to evaluate what we do, and become more in tune with our children.** This book will help caregivers weed out the confusing parenting advice and popular opinion out there from what is really in our children's best interest.

I will for sure be using the parenting workouts in this book with myself and with my clients.

Jill Osborne, EDS, LPC, CPCS, RPTS
Author of *Sam Feels Better Now! An Interactive Story for Children*

What kind of parent do you want to be? Kenley's book, *Pilates for Parenting* is an excellent resource for parents. With the problematic distractions children often face, parents need to be as diligent as possible. I love the creative idea of incorporating the Pilates structure with parenting advice. Kenley discusses the importance of showing up with a purpose and process so that your children feel loved and respected for who they are. *Pilates For Parenting* reminds us that every child deserves to have a parent who is well, child-focused, and a safe harbor. Readers are provided with excellent exercises to be proactive and thoughtful as you think through what makes sense for your family. **I recommend** *Pilates for Parenting***! It is a must-read for any parent or guardian. The ideas will help you take your parenting to the next level.**

Cathy Taughinbaugh, Certified Parent Coach
Founder of CathyTaughinbaugh.com

Pilates For Parenting

Stretch Yourself and Strengthen Your Family

Holli Kenley

Loving Healing Press

Ann Arbor, MI

Library of Congress Cataloging-in-Publication Data
Names: Kenley, Holli, 1951- author.
Title: Pilates for parenting : stretch yourself and strengthen your family
  / Holli Kenley.
Description: Ann Arbor, MI : Loving Healing Press, [2019] | Includes
  bibliographical references and index. | Summary: "Kenley models her
  exercises for improving parenting habits by analogy to the work of
  Joseph Pilates' method of physical therapy. In this system, parents are
  encouraged to stretch their levels of responsibility and causality in
  specific ways in service of improving the safety, nurturing, mentoring,
  and quality of life for their children"-- Provided by publisher.
Identifiers: LCCN 2019043642 (print) | LCCN 2019043643 (ebook) | ISBN
  9781615994885 (hardcover) | ISBN 9781615994878 (paperback) | ISBN
  9781615994892 (kindle edition) | ISBN 9781615994892 (epub)
Subjects: LCSH: Parenting. | Parent and child. | Pilates method.
Classification: LCC HQ755.8 .K4466 2019 (print) | LCC HQ755.8 (ebook) |
  DDC 306.874--dc23
LC record available at https://lccn.loc.gov/2019043642
LC ebook record available at https://lccn.loc.gov/2019043643

Published by
Loving Healing Press
5145 Pontiac Trail
Ann Arbor, MI 48105

www.LHPress.com
ino@LHPRess.com
Tollfree USA/CAN: 888-761-6268
FAX 734-663-6861

ISBN 978-1-61599-487-8 paperback
ISBN 978-1-61599-488-5 hardcover
ISBN 978-1-61599-489-2 eBook

Contents

We must become the people we want our children to be.

Joseph Chilton Pearce

Acknowledgments

Alexis, you bless me every day with the privilege of being a parent.

Dan, from the beginning you believed in me and in my promise of being a purposeful one.

A Heart Check

I have had the pleasure of knowing thousands of parents and guardians during my career as a teacher and therapist. There have been hundreds who were dedicated, involved, caring, nurturing, and who worked hard being the best at parenting. There were countless others whom I admired and respected, especially when it meant making some tough calls during difficult times. There were dozens of parents and guardians who sacrificed so their children would have more opportunities in life than they did. There are many stories I could share, but there is one mom who comes to mind who implemented a simple, tender, loving practice into her routine each night which embodies the essence of "Pilates For Parenting."

Rebekah is an extremely busy mom with four children under the age of twelve. Her days begin early, tending to each of her children's needs: five year old Jake, eight year old Lauren, ten year old Jordon, and eleven year old Alisa. As the children complete their morning rituals, Rebekah checks in with her husband, coordinating his work schedule with the children's various commitments: sports practices and games, theatrical rehearsals and performances, faith-based groups and classes, community activities, and other school-related responsibilities. In addition to all the demands on her schedule, Rebekah is Parent-Teacher Association (PTA) President at her children's elementary school. When she finds some "me time", Rebekah is a talented free-lance writer for a local magazine.

One afternoon on a warm summer day, Rebekah and I met in my home to collaborate on an article. During the two hours we worked, her four children quietly entertained themselves in the living room reading books and coloring. Several times, they asked permission to go outside where they played in the yard. As we were finishing up, I thought about Rebekah, her children, and her gentle patient approach to parenting. Over the years of observation, it was obvious she had a unique, special connection with each child.

Straightening up the notes and materials on the dining room table, I commented to Rebekah, "Your kids are remarkable. Your children have such a strong sense of themselves and yet each is unusually giving and kind."

Rebekah smiled, "Thank you, Holli."

I asked, "Although you are incredibly involved in and dedicated to your children's wellbeing, I'm wondering if there is any one practice, or ritual, or routine you implement which you feel makes a difference in your parenting and thus with each one of them?"

Rebekah chuckled as she spoke. "Our lives are crazy busy. Hectic most days!" Rebekah's demeanor turned serious but calm. "I do spend one on one time with each one of my children every day. Sometimes, it is just twenty or thirty minutes which is not a lot, but it is still important to do so. However, every night as I tuck each child into bed, I do what I call a "Heart Check."

The words, "Heart Check" grabbed me. I waited for Rebekah's explanation.

As I cuddle up, one at a time, next to my children, I place my head on their chest so one ear is listening to their heart. Then, I ask a few questions such as…. *How is your heart feeling? What does your heart want to say to me? What makes your heart happy? What makes it sad? How could I help to make your heart feel better?* And so on…." Rebekah's voice lowered. "This little ritual means so much to my kids, and it does to me."

Moved by Rebekah's words and with the visual of the "Heart Check" replaying in my mind, I responded, "What a safe and yet intimate way to connect with each child. What meaningful and critical messages of worth you are sending to Jake, Lauren, Jordon, and Alisa. They matter. Their feelings matter. They are important."

Rebekah's eyes watered as did mine. She added, "It takes so little time, and yet, it makes such a difference."

As we get ready to embrace "Pilates For Parenting", I'd like to do a "Heart Check" with you. As you think about your parenting, how is your heart feeling? What does your heart want to say? What makes your heart happy or sad? What would make your heart feel better?

While you reflect on those questions, I hope you'll be encouraged by Rebekah's words, "It takes so little time, and yet, it makes such a difference."

Welcome to "Pilates For Parenting"

What Is Pilates?

Pilates or Physical Mind Method, is a series of low-impact exercises designed by Joseph Pilates to develop *strength, flexibility, balance, and inner awareness.* Exercises which are low-impact are considered gentle workouts; they do not wear down or compromise healthy parts of the body. However, make no bones about it, while Pilates moves target the core, the exercises benefit other areas of the body as well. Founder and instructor of Black Girl Pilates Sonja Herbert states, "Pilates is a full-body exercise method that will help you do everything better" (*Self*, 2019).

Wouldn't it be great if you could apply these concepts to parenting?! Well, you can. Although you are not training to run a marathon, you do need to target your parental core—gently, consistently, thoroughly, and for the long haul – so your children will reap the benefits of your Parenting Workout.

What Can I Expect?

For those of you who are parents already, embracing a "Pilates For Parenting" approach is going to *strengthen* the effective parenting practices you already have in place, and it may *stretch* you in ways you had not thought of. It most likely will cause you to *flex* your parenting attitudes and approaches and to achieve a *balance* within your homes which will serve you and your children well. For our current parents *and* for anyone who is considering the idea of parenthood, the principles shared will challenge your thinking in positive and productive ways. It is our goal to raise your level of *inner awareness* when it comes to implementing healthy roles and tackling the heavy responsibilities of being a parent.

Pilates Self-Assessment and Pacing Guide

Because we are focusing on the most critical concepts of strengthening the parent-child relationship and because there are a plethora of exercises to complete within each chapter, it is vital you pace yourself. Also, the Warm Up and the Workouts have been placed in order of importance, targeting strategic areas which build onto the next. Therefore, to get the most out of "Pilates For Parenting," do not rush through the exercises simply to move on to the next area of focus. Spend as much time as you need on each exercise. Typically, it takes about twenty-one days to integrate a new behavior so that it becomes part of you and your routine.

To assist you, at the end of each chapter you will be provided with a Pilates Pacing Guide. You will assess your levels of success as well as areas which need more attention and time. And, most importantly, you will know if you are ready to move on to the next workout or not.

Are you ready to Stretch Yourself and Strengthen Your Family? Let's get started with Warm Up: I Matter and My Children Matter.

Pilates Warm Up: I Matter and My Children Matter

During the past ten years of writing and speaking about cyber bullying and screen dependence, the most important audience to reach is parents. Yes, the audience who matters the most is You—Parents and Guardians. Yes, You Matter. Do you really know how much?

From the moment your child is born or you become the guardian or parent of a child, your life changes. You no longer are the center of your universe. Your partner, spouse, or the father/mother of your child is no longer the most significant person in your life. Why?

Because, your child just made you the most important person in his life.

This is important.

Your child just made you the most important person in his life.

Your child's life depends on you. From the beginning stages of providing basic needs to the later stages of young adulthood when they leave the parental nest and begin their own lives, your children need you and deserve to have the best of you. Often times, parents and guardians begin their parenting with a strong commitment and steady involvement in their children's lives. As their children enter into middle and high school, they often back off or become less engaged. Emotions frequently expressed are, "My children just don't need me as much." Other times, with more children coming into the family or as other challenges arise, parents grow tired, stressed, and over-worked, not only neglecting their commitment to parenting but rationalizing it in the process. And, as societies have embraced technology to meet their needs for communication and social interaction, parents and guardians as well as their children are immersed in their own social interests, unknowingly becoming increasingly isolated and detached from one another.

Whether your family is in a strong place of connection or whether it needs some strengthening, we begin your Warm Up by developing your inner awareness around the importance of being parents or guardians. As you do so, let's not think about this process as something you have to do. Let's reframe it as this is something you get to do. After all, being a parent or guardian is an awesome privilege.

Let's begin with the first part of our Warm Up.

We are going to start with a simple but super important exercise. As is true with any new exercise, you must start with the right mindset. Regardless of the age of your children, begin each day with your first Pilates Warm Up.

Pilates Warm Up #1: I Matter To My Children

On a card or piece of paper, write down the following:

> **I Matter To My Children**
> - My children depend on me for their basic needs.
> - My children need my love and nurturance.
> - My attitudes, behaviors, and words influence or impact their lives.

1. Place this on your bathroom mirror or somewhere you will see it every morning.

2. As you are getting ready, read aloud and repeat this phrase at least three times, "I Matter To My Children."

3. After reflecting on its significance, read and repeat the next statements aloud, at least three times.

   - My children depend on me for their basic needs.
   - My children need my love and nurturance.
   - My attitudes, behaviors, and words influence and impact their lives.

4. Allow yourself time to take in the importance of their implications.

5. If you experience any negativity, guilt, or self-blame, let go of it.

6. Before you leave the room, repeat aloud one more time, "I Matter To My Children."

Remember, in this first Warm Up, you are cultivating an inner awareness of your importance as parents and guardians. This takes time. Be patient with yourself. As you move through our series "Pilates for Parenting," you will address specific areas of parenting where you will stretch yourself and strengthen your family.

As we continue to Warm Up, let's challenge ourselves a bit further.

From birth until your precious beings are launched into adulthood, you—in your roles as parents and guardians- will remain the most important and influential persons in your children's lives. Everything you do and say will impact your children. Everything you don't do and don't say will impact them. Wow! That's a lot to take in. But do take it in.

This is important.

Children learn about themselves from their primary caregivers and their environments. Parents and guardians who demonstrate a healthy responsibility for taking care of their children will find their children develop a positive identity and sense of self. When parents or guardians do not fulfill their roles or abuse/neglect their duties as caregivers, children form a fractured sense of self and feel a loss of identity and worth. In more extreme cases, children who feel abandoned or left to parent themselves fail to develop a healthy sense of attachment. Therefore, an excellent exercise to incorporate into your "Pilates For Parenting: Warm Up" is to check in daily with your children and see if they feel like they matter. And why they do or do not.

Pilates Warm Up #2: Do My Children Feel Like They Matter?

Age appropriately, each day when you have quiet alone time with your children or when you tuck your children in at night, spend a few minutes asking them the following questions.

As you do so, remember the following: Be still. Be patient. Be a good listener.

1. Do you feel important? Do you feel valuable? Do you feel like you matter? Why or why not?

2. On a scale of 1 -10 (10 being the highest), how much do you feel like you matter? Why?

3. What can I do or not do as your mom, dad, etc. which would help you to feel more valuable?

Parents and guardians, even though you may not be prepared to hear what your children have to say, your best report card on how you are doing is how they are doing. Give your children time to respond. If they are quiet, be still and wait. When they begin to share, listen to them. Listen intently. Do not react or become defensive. This is about your children; not about you. Comfort, nurture, and reassure them. Commit to implementing the following on a daily and nightly basis:

After your children have responded, implement the following.

1. Tell your children they matter, they are valuable, and they are important.

2. Tell them why.

3. Then, show them. Recall how Rebekah did her "Heart Check" each night and spent meaningful time, one on one, with each of her children every day. Follow her lead.

As you begin to shift your attitudes, behaviors, and words towards your children, remember these vulnerable beings are resilient and flexible. They welcome change a lot easier and better than we do. As you continue to stretch and grow, don't beat yourself up or lather on any guilt for regrets or mistakes. If needed, forgive yourself and ask your children for their forgiveness. Then, release any negativity and remind yourself that any exercise program takes time to internalize and to reap the benefits of its implementation.

Pilates Routine: Begin each day with "Pilates Warm Up #1: I Matter To My Children". In addition, schedule in time during the day and evening for "Pilates Warm Up #2: Do My Children Feel They Matter?" As you recommit yourself every day to embracing this mindset and routine, give yourself permission to put your inner awareness to work by developing a stronger sense of mattering for yourself and for your children.

Anytime we implement a new routine or work on changing a behavior, we can feel frustration. In order to keep a pulse on your progress and provide a safe space to express your feelings, it is strongly recommended to keep a parenting journal. You'll look back at it later and be glad you did.

Suggested Activity: Select a specific day and time at the end of each week and spend a few minutes journaling about your Warm Up exercises.

- What is going well?

- What has been a struggle? Why?

- What changes are you noticing, in your children and in yourself?

- What are you learning about your children and about yourself?

Self-Assessment and Pacing Guide

In the Welcome, you were introduced to the concept of a Self- Assessment and Pacing Guide. It is now time to conduct an honest assessment of your progress. Take a few moments, read over the criteria, and determine if you are ready or not to move forward.

Green Light: I have been implementing daily Warm Up Exercises #1 and #2 for three weeks. I feel confident with both exercises. I feel a change in myself and I see how my children are responding. They look forward to our one on one time as I check in with each of them, daily or nightly. I look forward to it also.
Move on to Workout #1.

Red Light: I haven't done anything or I've done very little with the daily Warm Ups. I'm ready now to recommit to daily Warm Ups #1 and #2, each for twenty-one consecutive days before moving on to Workout #1.

You will find Warm Ups #1 and #2 below.

Warm Up #1: I Matter To My Children

1. On a card or piece of paper, write down the words, " I Matter To My Child."

2. Place this on your bathroom mirror or somewhere you will see it every morning.

3. As you are getting ready, read loud and repeat the phrase three times.

4. As you are saying the phrase, remind yourself about its implications: Read aloud and repeat the following three times.

   - My children depend on me for their basic needs.

- My children need my love and nurturance.

- My attitudes, behaviors, and words influence and impact their lives.

5. As you finish getting ready for your day, let go of any negativity, guilt, or self-blame.

6. Before you leave the room, repeat aloud one more time, "I Matter To My Children."

Pilates Warm Up #2: Do My Children Feel Like They Matter?

Ask you children each of the following questions. Be still. Be patient. Be a good listener.

1. Do you feel important? Do you feel valuable? Do you feel like you matter? Why or why not?

2. On a scale of 1-10 (10 being the highest), how much do you feel like you matter? Why?

3. What can I do or not do as your mom, dad, etc. which would help you to feel more valuable?

After your children have responded, implement the following.

1. Tell your children they matter, they are valuable, and they are important.

2. Tell them why.

3. Then, show them. Recall how Rebekah did her "Heart Check" each night and spent meaningful time, one on one, with each of her children every day. Follow her lead.

Pilates Workout #1:
Am I Present Each and Every Day?

We are diving into a very important exercise regime – "Pilates For Parenting." Remember, by beginning your daily routine with Warm Ups #1 and #2, you are cultivating and cementing your mindset to be child-centered. One of benefits of Pilates exercises is when you start to stretch your inner-core by reframing your mindset, it will strengthen other areas of the parent-child relationship. As you continue to grow by integrating three workouts into "Pilates For Parenting," you will find there will be areas where you are doing well, others which need strengthening or improving, and there may be areas which need serious attention. Again, whatever the case, don't beat yourself up or give up. As with any exercise program, move slowly but keep moving.

Pilates Workout #1: Being Present

Working with young people both as a teacher and therapist and reflecting on many of the lessons learned from being a mother, I believe the most important practice to establish in the parent-child relationship is Being Present, or "showing up" for our children. As a researcher and author, the importance of how parents show up for their children was a critical finding in analyzing personal narratives obtained from a two year study: *Daughters Betrayed By Their Mothers: Moving From Brokenness To Wholeness* (2018). Although most parents and guardians equate this principle to the amount of time they spend with their children, we are speaking specifically to how you show up for your children or how present you are with your children. Yes, time is important; however, your capacity to fulfill your roles in healthy ways transcends quantity of time.

Let's take a look at three essential components as we begin "Workout #1: Being Present"

- Stability and Wellness
- Selflessness and Child-Focused
- Stillness and Being A Safe Harbor

Let's get started!

Stability and Wellness

To be present for your children, you must be stable. You must be well: emotionally, psychologically, and physically. In order for parents and guardians to be able to meet their children's needs, they must be not be consumed by their own. It is not uncommon for children's needs to be over-looked or for them to be severely neglected when parents and guardians are suffering from untreated or unresolved issues, including but not limited to the following:

- Substance addiction

- Behavioral addictions such a gambling, gaming, and pornography

- Clinical disorders such as Depression, Anxiety, Post Traumatic Stress Disorder, and Bi Polar Disorder

- Other disorders which present themselves in our personalities such as Narcissistic, Borderline, and Histrionic features

- Past childhood trauma, abuse, and neglect

- Engagement in dangerous relationships (past and present)

In addition to clinical, personality, and relational issues, there are a plethora of unforeseen and uncontrollable circumstances which tragically compromise the healthy functioning of parents and guardians. A few examples include:

- Individuals who are suffering from life-threatening diseases

- Individuals who are victims of unspeakable injustices, forms of oppression, and environmental disasters, etc.

- Military personnel who have served their countries bravely and who have sustained life-altering injuries

What is important is how parents and guardians respond to these challenges and to their responsibilities in parenting. Committed and caring parents and guardians actively work recovery programs and implement healing practices in managing their illnesses, diseases, and disorders. While these adults are courageously battling to improve their wellbeing, they are working simultaneously toward increasing their capacity to show up for their children. Within the context of our discussion regarding stability and wellness, we are talking about the following condition.

When addictions or other unhealthy behaviors take on a life of their own, parents and guardians cannot be present for their children.

This is essential. Read it again.

When addictions or other unhealthy behaviors take on a life of their own, parents and guardians cannot be present for their children.

In my private practice working with adults raised in highly dysfunctional environments, I have found that many of my clients' parents and guardians suffered from clinical issues such as addiction, depression, and Post Traumatic Stress Disorder. Their parents' capacities to be present for their children was additionally compromised by the presence of personality disorders. Recently, one client painfully described how her bi-polar, narcissistic mother was unable to "mother her" in the ways she needed. She detailed how the roles within her household were reversed, "It was upside down in my home. I had to take care of my mother."

It is quite common for children to take on parental roles when adults within the home are unwilling to fulfill them or they are incapable of doing so. The ramifications of this are long-lasting and quite complex. For the purposes of "Pilates For Parenting," we want to focus on preventing this by helping parents to identify their areas of wellness while acknowledging and addressing areas which need work.

You will begin Workout #1 by assessing your levels of stability and wellness. This requires you to conduct an honest self-inventory. This is difficult; therefore, I encourage you to take your time. Pause and take a few deep breaths as needed. First, begin thinking about the following three questions and how you would answer them.

Stability and Wellness Questions

- Am I stable?

- Am I well: physically, emotionally, and psychologically?

- Am I taking care of my needs at the expense of my children's?

Then, either in a journal, or on your laptop, or whatever writing modality is comfortable for you, describe how you are showing up for your children. Spend as much time as needed. This exercise is extremely important.

Plates Workout #1: Exercise #1 – Stability and Wellness

1. First, identify behaviors which demonstrate your stability and wellness. These are actions which illustrate the positive healthy ways in which you are taking care of your children. Write down as many as you can think of. This is a time to focus in on what you are doing well. For example:
   - I am fully employed so that I can provide for my children.
   - I prepare meals for my children.
   - I make sure their basic needs for clothing and shelter are met.
   - I provide structure and routine for my children.

2. Secondly, identify behaviors which require change. Also, write down three action steps to address each behavior needing improvement. For example:
   - Behavior: I need to spend more time with my children.

- Action steps: I will involve my children in the preparation and cleanup of meals. We will eat dinner together. I will spend one on one time with each child before or after dinner.

3. Lastly, identify behaviors which need to be eliminated. Also write down three action steps which will move you towards achieving this goal. For example:

   - Behavior: I will stop meeting up with my friends every day after work to socialize.

   - Action steps: I will make a commitment to myself and my children that I will be home immediately after work. I will communicate to my friends that I am readjusting my priorities; my children come first. I will turn to a healthy friend or mentor for accountability and check in weekly.

Pilates Workout #1 is one of the most challenging exercises and yet its potential for strengthening your family is huge. Spend as much time on this as needed. However, don't take on too much at once, especially with behaviors you want to change or eliminate. Begin with one behavior you want to change and one you want to eliminate. Think through your three action steps for each one. Make sure they are realistic and achievable. If you find they are not working, revisit your action steps and revise them. With "Pilates For Parenting," you have permission to fall short as long as you self-assess and then recommit to your goals.

Once you have maintained a healthier routine consistently for at least three weeks, then add a new behavior to change or eliminate. Make sure you acknowledge the areas in which you feel you are doing well and add those to your first list of healthy behaviors. If you are discovering there are issues which require professional services for intervention, treatment, and support, seek out appropriate resources and make a commitment to a recovery program or process.

Remember, in order to give your children your best, you must be your best.

Selflessness and Child-Focused

In order to be fully present for your children, you must first be stable and well. As we have discussed, if you are consumed with unhealthiness in its various forms, you navigate from a very self-centered and self-serving position. Getting your needs met becomes a priority, not your children's. Although the second component in Workout #1: Selflessness and Child-Focused relates to Stability and Wellness, it deserves special attention.

Over the past several years, we have been experiencing a behavioral shift where young people and adults alike are becoming more self-absorbed and self-focused. This is understandable. As we have moved into a technologically-driven culture to meet our social and relational needs, we have become much more egocentric, constantly self-promoting and seeking self-validation through various social networking platforms. In order to be present with our children, we must acknowledge the energy and resources we spend on screen distractions such as cell phones, gaming, texting, etc. In researching *Power Down & Parent Up* (2016), tweens to teens reported how they wished their parents would spend less time on their technology. When you demonstrate your capacity for selflessness and turn away from self-indulgent behaviors, you show your children they are more important than your phones, emails, texts, tweets, posts, games, etc. You show them they matter.

Technology is not the only area of concern. There are other interests, pursuits, or pastimes which detract from being Child-Focused; for example: work, sports, hobbies, relationships. This too is understandable. However, when your harmonious passions become obsessive ones, you stray from being present for your children. In other words, a new pastime or passion may start out as an innocent way to escape, have fun, or unwind. You are drawn to repeating the behavior because it enhances your life and brings harmony into it. Unfortunately, over time and with increased access, exposure, or consumption, your new escape can become an obsession, consuming your attention and taking it away from your children.

Remember, as we embrace our Pilates Workouts, we are not saying you must eliminate the pleasures in your life. You are seeking balance as you improve your parenting. Let's keep striving for a healthy equilibrium.

As you did with the first exercise, think and reflect on the following question. Don't rush this. Be truthful with yourself as you stretch and flex your parenting skills.

Selflessness and Child-Focused Questions

- Is the attention I give to a device, project, place, job, interest, hobby, game, etc. greater than, equal to, or less than the attention I give to my children?

Pilates Workout #1: Being Present Exercise #2 – Selflessness and Child-Focused

As you did before, conduct an honest self-inventory of how child-focused you are. In ways which are convenient and comfortable, write down your responses to the following three areas.

1. First, identify behaviors which demonstrate how, when, and where you give attention to your children. This is a time to brag and boast. Don't be shy. For example:

   - When I come home from work, I check in with each child, face to face, for at least five minutes.

   - My son and I play catch at least three times a week.

   - I help my daughter with her homework every night.

2. Secondly, name behaviors which require change and write down three action steps. For example:

- Behavior: I need to cut way back on my video gaming.

- Action steps: I will talk to my children about my video game habit and how I realize it is taking time away from them. I will put away all video games until the weekend. I will limit my play to one hour on the weekend and schedule it during our family tech time.

3. Thirdly, identify behaviors or actions which need to be eliminated and delineate three action steps. It is only natural to be defensive or in denial about some of our behaviors and their impact on our children. If you find yourself minimizing or rationalizing a habit, pastime, or interest, ask your children how they feel about the time you spend away from them. Take a deep breath. If we ask them for their input, we must be prepared to listen and respond accordingly. For example:

- Behavior: I'm always on my phone. I'm never without it. Even when I'm at home, I tell my kids I need it for work, but I don't. My ten year old daughter says I am addicted.

- Action steps: I am going to put my phone away when I come home from work. I will not check it again until they are in bed. I going to talk to my children about the changes and model healthier tech behavior. If I need more support, I'm going to reach out for help.

Because we live in tech-driven societies, it is becoming a norm to pay more attention to our phones, laptops, iPads, screens, etc. than to our children and to one another. While technology is here to stay and it serves us in many incredible ways, you want to remain mindful of the importance of face to face connection and interaction. Most importantly, by looking into the eyes of your children, paying attention to them, and being fully present for them, you message them they matter.

If you need more support, consider picking up a copy of *Power Down & Parent Up* There are seven practical strategies and four guidelines for managing your technology and maintaining a healthy family. It's not about banning technology; it's about balancing it. And, it's about consistently showing up for your kids.

As we address each of the areas of Being Present, you may have noticed there is overlap in your behavioral inventories. If there is, this is important. It demonstrates how one area of concern or needed attention is impacting your parenting in multiple ways. Again, do not beat yourself up. Pay attention to it and work on it.

Stillness and Being a Safe Harbor

In order to show up for your kids or to be present fully for them, parents and guardians must also be Still. Being Still is not easy, especially in today's fast-paced culture. More importantly, being Still requires you first must be Stable and Selfless. This is important.

When you are stable and selfless for your children, you become their safe-harbor. *Read it again, aloud.*

When you are stable and selfless for your children, you become their safe-harbor.

As families face challenges and children confront theirs, parents have a choice about how they respond. Catastrophizing and dramatizing situations muddies the waters and creates unnecessary currents. Reacting with anger and criticism typically fuels the upheaval. Stable and well parents and guardians remain still, implementing rational and reasonable processes to move through the turbulence. Child-focused parents and guardians listen and communicate openly. Stable and selfless parents respond with calm and comfort. When parents and guardians provide a warm loving harbor for their children to tether themselves, children know they are safe, and they are more likely to turn to them when facing personal challenges.

Recently, I was talking with a mom, Anna, regarding her seventeen year old daughter Karina. Although they are quite close and communicate well, Anna has been frustrated with Karina around the lack of communication when Karina is out late with her friends. Anna expects Karina to text her if Karina decides to change plans, locations, or times. In their discussion, Karina became defensive, arguing how her mom was not trusting of her. Anna remained calm, explaining to her daughter it was not a lack of trust issue but a protective measure. Anna was relieved to report to me that by the end of their conversation, both Karina and she had a new understanding of one another's perspectives. Karina committed to texting her mom in future situations. Anna reaffirmed her trust in her daughter and in her appreciation for talking things through.

Although this example does not illustrate a present danger, it may help prevent a potential one. Parents and guardians often find themselves in frightening or critical situations because of the choices their children make or because of circumstances beyond their control. During these difficult times, emotions can and will run high. In implementing "Pilates For Parenting," you will continue to stretch yourself by increasing your inner awareness as to how you react to your children and how you can learn to respond more effectively. Let's keep growing.

Stillness and Being a Safe Harbor Questions

As you have done previously, reflect on the following questions:

- Am I a safe harbor for my children? Why or why not?

- Do I take time to be still? Do I react or do I respond?

Spend as much time as you need on this. For clarification, as noted there are times of crisis or upset when parents and guardians fly off the handle or over-react to circumstances or situations. Heightened emotions are characteristic of parents and guardians who are fearful for their children's safety and wellbeing. However, these reactive behaviors should not be the norm or a default emotion. Thus, when assessing your levels of stillness, ask yourself if your behaviors reflect a consistent pattern of calm and compassion, or if they are representative of an ongoing display of anger and aggression.

Once again, conduct an honest self-inventory of the areas listed below. Write down your responses in your journal, on your laptop, or in whatever ways you find comfortable.

Pilates Workout #1: Being Present Exercise #3 - Stillness and Being a Safe Harbor

1. First, identify behaviors which demonstrate evidence of being a safe harbor for your children. For example:

   - My children tell me they can talk to me about anything.

   - I have clear guidelines for my children and they have responsibilities. However, we talk over what is working for our family, what is not, and we make adjustments when needed.

   - I monitor my children's behaviors, online and off, but I do so with respect.

2. Secondly, name behaviors which require change and list three action steps.

   - Behavior: I need to listen more to my children. I'm great at giving advice, but they say I don't listen.

   - Action steps: When we talk, we all need to put away our phones because no one is listening. I will not interrupt my children when they are talking. I will ask them how I can help and I will problem-solve with them, if they need me to.

3. Thirdly, identify behaviors which need to be eliminated and write down three action steps:

   - Behavior: I need to get control of my anger. It frightens my kids.

   - Action steps: I will acknowledge my anger and apologize to my children. I will get help. I will make an appointment to see a counselor. I also know of an anger management group that a friend of mine attends. I will go with him.

As you think about Being Present, it is important to recognize what we have discussed is not easy stuff. It is hard to self-reflect and self-assess, especially when it comes to behaviors which are deeply engrained. We tend to feel enormous shame when we recognize these behaviors are not healthy and may indeed be hurting our children. Remember these things:

1. No one is a perfect parent. No one.

2. It is never too late to regroup and start again. Never.

3. Parents and guardians, You Matter. Yes, You Matter.

4. Parents and guardians, Your Children Matter. Yes, Your Children Matter.

For now, take a deep breath. Release any guilt or other negative thoughts or feelings.

Pilates Routine: As you continue to flex and strengthen your parenting skills, focus on one or two behaviors at a time which need changing or eliminating. When we take on too much at once, we usually give up because it feels overwhelming or defeating. As you begin to feel success or improvement in one or two areas, think about adding another. However, as you might have already discovered, as you address one area of concern, the assigned exercises also tend to mitigate other areas of vulnerability. That is why "Pilates For Parenting" is so cool!

Suggested Activity: Take out your journal. As you begin implementing Pilates Workout #: 1 Being Present exercises, at the end of each week select a day and time and respond to the following prompts.

• What am I learning about Being Present for my children?

• What is coming easily? What is working well?

• Which of the three behaviors of Being Present has been the most challenging to change or eliminate: Stability, Selflessness, or Stillness? Why? What additional action steps will I commit to?

Self-Assessment and Pacing Guide

It is time once again to conduct an honest assessment of your progress. Take a few moments, read over the criteria, and determine if you are ready or not to move forward.

Green Light: I have continued with daily Warm Ups #1 and #2. In addition, in each of the three areas of Workout #1 Being Present, I have identified positive behaviors, and I have targeted negative behaviors which need to be changed or eliminated. I have implemented actions steps in each of the areas needing work for a minimum of three weeks. I feel confident in my progress. My children have given me positive feedback. Move on to Workout #2.

Red Light: I have fallen short in meeting my commitments in the daily Warm Ups. I need to stop, go back, and recommit to them before moving on.

Although I have maintained my commitments in the daily Warm Ups, I haven't done anything or I've done very little in Workout #1. I'm ready now to recommit to Pilates Workout #1 Being Present Exercises #1, #2, and #3. I will identify positive behaviors. For each behavior which needs changing or eliminating, I will work three or more action steps for twenty-one consecutive days before adding another area of concern. I realize this may take me months to do. I'm committed for however long it takes.. You'll find Exercises #1, #2, and #3 below.

Pilates Workout #1: Exercise #1 - Stability and Wellness

Questions to reflect upon:
- Am I stable?
- Am I well: physically, emotionally, and psychologically?
- Am I taking care of my needs at the expense of my children's?

Describe how you are showing up for your children.
1. First, identify behaviors which demonstrate your stability and wellness.
2. Secondly, identify behaviors which require change. Write down three action steps.
3. Lastly, identify behaviors which need to be eliminated. Write down three action steps.

Pilates Workout #1: Exercise #2 - Selflessness and Child-Focused

Question to reflect upon:
- Is the attention I give to a device, project, job, interest, hobby, game, etc. greater than, equal to, or less than the attention I give to my children?

Conduct an honest inventory. Identify behaviors which are working well and those which need work.
1. First, identify behavior which demonstrate how, when, and where you give attention to your children.
2. Secondly, name the behaviors which require change and write down three action steps.
3. Thirdly, identify behaviors or actions which need to be eliminated and delineate three action steps to address them.

Pilates Workout #1: Exercise #3 - Stillness and Being A Safe Harbor

Questions to reflect upon:
- Am I a safe harbor for my children? Why or why not?
- Do I take time to be still? How do I respond?

Conduct an honest inventory. Identify behaviors which are working and those which need attention.

1. First, identify behaviors which demonstrate evidence of being a safe harbor for your children.

2. Secondly, identify behaviors which require change and list three action steps.

3. Thirdly, identify behaviors which need to be eliminated and write down three action steps

Pilates Workout #2:
Am I Doing What Is Best or What is Easy or Popular?

In our "Pilates For Parenting" workout regime, Being Present was placed first because it is the most fundamental practice to put into place. This is important.

Growing your parent-child relationship is dependent upon your capacity to be well, to be child-focused, and to be a safe harbor for your children.

Read again, aloud.

Growing your parent-child relationship is dependent upon your capacity to be well, to be child- focused, and to be a safe harbor for your children.

The three areas of Being Present take a great deal of work. As we add workouts to your routine, continue to begin each day with your Warm Ups and Workout #1. These exercises are not a one and done. They are ongoing. If you are feeling a bit over-whelmed, recall how the best way to change or improve behavior is to take small steps, achieve your goal, and then move forward. If you have a setback, readjust your goals and begin again. Don't give up. Recommit yourself each and every day. Celebrate the rewards of growing the parent-child relationship.

Let's move on with "Pilates Workout #2 – Protecting"

Today's workout may seem like common sense. Of course, parents and guardians should protect their children. However, because of all the changes and challenges parents and guardians face every day, there are two areas which can help us to do a better job of Protecting our children:

- Safety
- Nurturance

Safety

In order to protect your children, you need to focus on their safety. You must be pro-active about who or what you allow into their lives, and when and where. Keeping your children safe means the following:

Doing what is best for my children's health and wellbeing –not what is easy or popular.

This is critically important. Keeping your children safe means:

Doing what is best for my children's health and wellbeing- not what is easy or popular.

In today's technologically-driven culture, some of the most heartbreaking stories from parents and guardians involve the dangers of the Internet. Whether it is cyber bullying, revenge porn, predators, etc., children are being targeted, victimized, and placed in high-risk situations. And yet, frequently when parents or guardians are questioned about their guidelines for safe practices regarding their children's usage or if they have a "Family Media Plan" (see Appendix A) in place, many have no response.

When I am speaking to audiences, parents and guardians are surprised to learn that before we turn over any piece of technology to any age child, we must be willing to do the hard work up front. This requires we find out what the risks are as well as the benefits. We need to know how to implement practices and establish expectations for their usage which will minimize the dangers and educate us on how to intervene if the unthinkable happens. This safety issue is fully addressed in *Power Down & Parent Up: Cyber Bullying, Screen Dependence, and Raising Tech-Healthy Children* (2016). Parents and guardians, *Power Down & Parent Up* is a concise thirty-two pages but powerful resource just for you. It is a roadmap which will serve as a guide down a path of safety as you and your children navigate the cyber landscape.

Several years ago while speaking to an audience on cyber bullying, a parent raised her hand and asked, "Holli, do I have a right to invade my child's privacy? Should I be checking her texts or other social networking accounts?"

My response was compassionate yet firm. "We have a responsibility to protect our children. And, I will show you how to do so with respect and regard for them." After demonstrating to the audience how to implement a "Family Media Plan" (see Appendix A), there was relief on their faces.

Technology issues are important; however, with any social behavior, parents and guardians should always keep their children's safety in mind when making decisions about their degree of access and exposure to, or consumption of anything.

As you get ready to begin Pilates Workout #2- Protecting, stretch yourself with an important parenting principle: by doing the hard work upfront, it may save you from heartache in the end.

Let's keep growing.

Safety Questions

In embracing a Pilates regimen, your exercises are meant to focus in on areas which need strengthening. Therefore, in order for you to be purposeful about protecting your children, you must we must be willing to ask and answer several essential questions regarding your decision-making and your children's safety.

Read over the following Safety Questions. Spend a few minutes reflecting on them.

1. How much do I know about this person, place, thing, activity, etc.? Have I done my research, conducted background checks, or consulted with trusted knowledgeable sources? What have I learned?

2. Why am I agreeing to this? Why am I disagreeing?

3. How will this benefit my children? How will it not?

4. Am I willing to commit to monitoring, supervising, or following-up with this person, place, or thing, etc.? Am I willing to explore my children's degree of involvement and how they are being affected or impacted? If so, what will that commitment and follow-up exploration look like?

By applying these questions to your decision-making process, you will not only be able to make an informed decision but you will also be able to explain your reasoning to your children. Let's take a look at an example.

In speaking to audiences about technology, I am often asked what the appropriate age is for children to be on social networking sites. In sharing my recommendations, I move through the criteria listed above.

First, I ask them to consider the advice of reliable sources and expert opinions. For example:

- Most sites recommend or require users to be at least age 13.

- Most health care advocates who are knowledgeable about cognitive develop-ment and social risks recommend age 15 and over.

I also ask them to do their own research and discover what experts are recom-mending. (see Appendix B - Resources)

Secondly, I ask parents and guardians to think about their reasons for allowing their children to be on social networking sites. For example:

- Are you caving into pressure from your children?

- Are you worried your children will feel left out?

- Are you thinking other parents or guardians will judge you?

It is critical to understand your motivations for making a decision or agreeing to something. I encourage parents and guardians to step away from the emotional pull of their children's reactions and to give themselves time to sort through their reasons before a decision is made.

Thirdly, I ask audiences to list the benefits and the costs of allowing their children to be on the social networking sites. For example:

- Benefits: children will have more friends; be more social; fit in with their peers.

- Costs: children might not understand the dangers; children might be cyber bullied. Children may become more isolated from family as they spend more time online.

Lastly, I ask parents and guardians what their commitment will look like in supervising, monitoring, or following up if they allow their children to join social networking sites. For example:

- Are you willing to write up a Family Media Plan, which includes children and adults, and to explain your expectations around the degree of usage and monitoring of all technology?

- Are you willing to sit down with your children and visit their net neighborhoods on a consistent basis?

Even after thoughtful decisions are made, circumstances can and will shift. As situations arise, be prepared to answer the "whys" around your decisions to your children. Avoid sayings such as, "Because I said so." Or, "Because I am the parent." If needed, ask questions of your children to obtain more information. Give yourself time to make a well-informed decision. Age appropriately, explain how you are making adjustments in your decision-making and why.

Let's get started with Exercise #1.

It is quite understandable how reading over and reflecting on the Safety Questions may illicit a few uncomfortable feelings. If so, take a deep breath. Pause and keep going. Others may feel a sense of pride in how they are approaching their decisions regarding safety. Remember, by becoming more aware of your parenting weaknesses and strengths, you continue to grow the parent-child relationship.

Pilates Workout #2: Protecting Exercise #1 - Safety

Think back to a recent decision you made regarding your children and respond to the Safety Questions. Write your answers down in your journal or in other ways which are comfortable for you.

1. How much did I know about this person, place, thing, activity, etc.? Did I do my research, conduct background checks, or consult with trusted knowledgeable sources? What did I learn?

2. Why did I agree to this? Why did I disagree?

3. How did this benefit my children? How did it not?

4. Did I commit to monitoring, supervising, or following-up with this person, place, or thing, etc.? Did I explore my children's degree of involvement and how they were being affected or impacted? If so, what did that commitment look like?

After responding to the safety questions in Exercise #1, return to your writing material and answer these follow-up questions:

- Which of the criteria did I use in making my decision?

- What did I learn from the decision-making process and from the outcome?

- What would I do differently next time?

- What worked well for my children and me?

One of the most remarkable characteristics of children is they are unusually forgiving and resilient. If you have made decisions which you now recognize are not in the best interest of your children's health and wellbeing, it is absolutely permissible to change your mind. Age appropriately, explain to them what you have learned and why you are making adjustments. Children respond well when parents and guardians take the time to explain their rationale.

Recently during a conversation with a friend who has a daughter in college and a son in middle school, she shared, "When my husband and I realize we've really blown it, we tell our kids, 'We made a mistake'! We care about you. We are going to do a redo!'" She laughed and added, "My kids are great about it They appreciate how we know we are not perfect and that we mess up too!"

Remember, it's never too late to do a redo. NEVER! Let's move on to Exercise #2.

In anticipation of a pending decision or if you are forecasting a redo on a current decision regarding your children, implement the next exercise.

Pilates Workout #2: Protecting Exercise #2 – Safety

Take your time. This process will set the tone for your future decision-making.

1. Identify a pending decision or a redo on a past decision regarding your children and their safety.

2. Utilizing the criteria in the Safety Questions, work through each of the questions as you process your decision.

3. Talk with your children about your decision. Referencing the Safety Questions, explain how and why you came to your decision.

4. Listen to your children's concerns. Answer their questions. Make adjustments as needed and as you gather more information.

5. Keep communication open between your children and you. Let them know how much they matter.

After you have implemented Exercise #2, reflect upon and respond to the following questions.

- How did this process work for you? For your children?

- What went well?

- What would you do differently next time?

- What are you learning as a family?

Parents and guardians, in today's unpredictable and unstable world, it is not easy to keep your children safe. You must remember you are their first line of defense. When you are vigilant about their protection, when you make the tough calls, and when you do so with comprehensive, compassionate, and caring rationale, you signal to your children they matter. Over time and with consistency, your children will believe, know, and trust they matter, and they will respond accordingly.

Let's move on to our second area of Protecting - Nurturance.

Nurturance

The second component to protecting our children is based around the principle of nurturance. Most of you are familiar with the word nurture. Although it is a gentle word, when applied to your "Pilates For Parenting" exercises, nurturance takes on a stronger and more sustainable connotation: the ability to care for over time. With its intentional application, you will not only fortify your parenting but your children will flourish because of it.

As you incorporate this aspect of protecting our children into our "Pilates For Parenting," strengthening your nurturing skills means the following:

Caring for your children over time, remaining cautious about detaching from them too early while being mindful of their need for independence and autonomy.

This is important. Read again, aloud. Strengthening your nurturing skills means the following:

Caring for your children over time, remaining cautious about detaching from them too early while being mindful of their need for independence and autonomy.

When speaking with parents and guardians about benefits of technology and nurturing your children, there is strong support for being able to stay in contact with them, checking in on their safety and caring for their needs. There is no denying in an age of terrorism and unspeakable acts of cruelty, technology provides you with a modicum of comfort with your accessibility to one another and emergency services. In addition, it is great to be able to communicate all sorts of random messages such as schedule changes, reminders for pick up times, and sharing words of encouragement and support. All of these parent-child communications signal to your children you care for them, over time and with their wellbeing in mind.

However, as dependence upon technology has increased for communication and social interaction, not just with friends and co-workers but within families, we are witnessing a shift in the psychological and social development of our children. While oversight and involvement in your children's lives is critical, unhealthy screen-attachment can sabotage the healthy development of autonomous identities and the construction of independent, self-sufficient young adults. A more thorough investigation of these consequences can be found in Dr. Jean Twenge's well-researched book, *iGen: Why Today's Super-Connected Kids Are Growing Up Less Rebellious, More Tolerant, Less Happy- and Completely Unprepared for Adulthood* (2017).

How then are you to protect your children while preparing them for adulthood? Let's take a look at the following metaphor and learn from it.

Although there are numerous creatures in the animal kingdom which provide us with lessons on how to be nurturing, deer are a perfect example. The adult doe instinctually protects her newborns while affording them brief moments of autonomy as they learn necessary survival skills. In the early months after birth, a mother doe stays extremely close to her babies. Although she is leading the way through the rocky terrain searching for food, she remains vigilant keeping a watchful eye on them and on any potential danger. Mother doe are also extraordinarily keen to the dangers of premature exposure to the wilderness, introducing survival elements and foreign environments slowly and cautiously. As her young fawn or buck mature, a mother doe will distance herself further in proximity from her young ones; however, it is clear how keeping them out of harm's way remains her first priority. At first sight, scent, or sound of an intruder, she signals their departure and secures their safety. As the seasons pass, the young adults saunter through unfamiliar terrain, cautious but confident on their own. Mother doe eyes them from afar, a distant protector and witness to the rewards of preparing them for adulthood.

Once again, in your "Pilates For Parenting," you are seeking a healthy balance in your roles as nurturers, protecting and preparing your children.

Let's continue to stretch ourselves. Parents and guardians, as you consider the deer metaphor, assess how you are providing nurturance for your children. Read over the following Nurturance Questions. Spend a few moments reflecting on them. Take your time.

Nurturance Questions

1. Do I watch over my children (using electronic monitoring and face-to-face supervision)? Do I know where they are, what they are doing, and with whom – in their net neighborhood and their real one?

2. Did I start out strong in my commitment to nurturance when my children were young and have I sustained that commitment over time? If so, in what ways? If not, what areas do I need to improve?

3. Have I exposed my children prematurely or allowed unsupervised access too early to a person, place, thing, etc., without considering their safety? Have I adequately prepared them with the appropriate insights and tools to handle potential dangers and possible harm? What areas do I need to address?

4. While caring for my children over time, am I being mindful of their needs for independence and autonomy? Am I encouraging them to make decisions on their own (age appropriately), to take on responsibilities, and to experience failure as well as success?

These questions are extremely important. Take your time as you think through them carefully before you respond. Remember, "Pilates For Parenting," like any worthwhile exercise program, can be uncomfortable at first as you stretch and strengthen areas you have not worked on before or areas you have overlooked. Also, remind yourself that you rarely, if ever, change anything when you are feeling cozy or comfortable in what you are doing. Give yourself permission to allow any guilt, doubt, or discomfort to motivate you to recommit and keep going.

In working with parents and guardians as a teacher and therapist, I have found that over the years most parents are very vigilant about Nurturance Question #1. However, as young children mature, other children enter the family, and with an abundance of hectic schedules accompanied with all kinds of stress, many parents and guardians begin to struggle with Nurturance Questions #2. As we discussed earlier in Being Present for your children, as your children become more independent and develop their identities, they still need your guidance and oversight.

Nurturance Question #3 addresses some of the most challenging areas of caring for your children over time. With access and exposure to and consumption of anything at your children's fingertips, harm is just a click away. With online social comparison in full force 24/7 and real life peer pressure still in play, your children struggle moment by moment to define and defend themselves. They are constantly faced with making responsible, rational, and reasonable decisions when their brains have not developed the capacity to do so. Because the pre-fontal cortex does not fully develop until the mid-twenties, children make decisions based on their emotions, feelings, and response to rewards. They are naturally impulsive and reactive. It is not their fault. Thus, without adequate structure, preparation, and supervision, parents and guardians often and un-knowingly place their children in high risk situations. Although your children's relationship with technology is an extremely important area of concern, the Nurturance Questions apply to all aspects of their lives.

For example, several months ago, I was working with an adult client who experienced ongoing trauma in her childhood. I will call her Emily. Because Emily's father abandoned the family when she was an adolescent and her mother was very low functioning, Emily referred to her siblings and herself as "free range kids," allowed to roam their neighborhoods and often placed in harm's way. Although Emily was the oldest and had a good head on her shoulders, she described her anxiety in trying to provide safety and care for herself and her siblings. At such a young age, Emily did not have the insights or tools to navigate parental roles nor was she prepared for such responsibilities.

Lastly, Nurturance Question #4 is tricky in finding a balance between protecting and preparing. Like the deer, it requires instinct, skill, and a keen understanding of the personalities and needs of each of your children. What works for one may not work for another. What is most important is you remain fully Present as learned in Workout #1, while nurturing your children into adulthood.

Pilates Workout #2: Protecting Exercise #3 – Nurturance

Let's get started implementing your Nurturance exercise.

Let's return to the Nurturance Questions. This parenting inventory is not an easy one. Take as much time as you need. Write down your responses in your journal or in ways which are comfortable for you. Refer back to Pilates Workout #2: Protecting Exercise #3 – Nurturance on page 31.

Within each question, there are multiple questions. Where applicable, answer "yes, no, or sometimes." Then provide at least two examples to support your answers on the remaining questions.

1. Do I watch over my children (using electronic monitoring and face to face supervision)? Do I know where they are, what they are doing, and with whom – in their net neighborhood and their real one? For example:

   - Yes, I watch over my children with face to face supervision. And I know where they are and what they are doing.
     1. We always keep a family calendar with our schedules on the refrigerator.
     2. We always text each other about our schedules, any changes, etc.

   - Sometimes, I check their electronic communications but I don't always know what they are doing online.
     1. I'm not sure who their online friends are.
     2. I don't know what they are posting on social networks.

2. Did I start out strong in my commitment to nurturance when my children were young and have I sustained that commitment over time? If so, in what ways? If not, what areas do I need to improve? For example:

   - Yes, in some areas I have maintained a strong commitment to nurturance.
     1. I have stayed actively involved in their schooling and their interests.
     2. As my children have matured, I still set aside time to talk to them about what is going on in their lives.

   - No, there are a couple of areas where I could improve.
     1. I need to learn more about their online friends. The more time my son spends online, the more lonely he is.
     2. With my teenage daughter, I don't feel we are connecting as much. I think she is pulling away from me. I'm not sure what to do.

3. Have I exposed my children prematurely or allowed unsupervised access too early to a person, place, thing, etc., without considering their safety? Have I

adequately prepared them with the appropriate insights and tools to handle potential dangers and possible harm? What areas do I need to address? For example:

- Yes and No. I think there are some areas which I have been very careful not to expose my children to but there are other areas I need to address.
    1. I monitor the kinds of videos and other media they watch.
    2. I don't know all the different social networking sites my children visit.
- Sometimes I have done a good job preparing them to handle potential dangers and possible harm, but I need to improve on this.
    1. I've talked to my children about taking photos of themselves and sharing them with strangers.
    2. I've talked about cyber bullying with my children, but I need to do a better job of helping them when they are victimized or if they see someone else who is.

4. While caring for my children over time, am I being mindful of their needs for independence and autonomy? Am I encouraging them to make decisions on their own(age appropriately), to take on responsibilities, and to experience failure as well as success? For example:

- Yes, I am aware that my children need their independence and I work on honoring that age appropriately.
    1. As my children demonstrate responsibility, I give them more leeway. If they come home on time, I am more likely to let them stay out later the next time.
    2. Before my children have free time, they must complete their homework and chores.
- Sometimes I encourage them to make their own decisions, but many times I rescue them because I don't want them to fail.
    1. I write false excuses for my child when she does not do her homework.
    2. I don't make my son go to baseball practice if he doesn't want to. I know this hurts him and his team.

After you have answered the Nurturance Questions and provided examples to support your findings, take a deep breath. Acknowledge both your strengths and weaknesses. Then, respond to the following:

- What is the most important area I need to work on?

  1. Write down one area of concern.

  2. Then, identify three action steps to address that area.

  3. Implement the actions steps for three weeks or until they are a part of your behavior before adding another. For example:

- Area of concern: Sometimes I encourage my children to make their own decisions, but many times I rescue them because I don't want them to fail.

  1. I will not lie for my children for any reason.

  2. I will make sure my children keep their word once they have made a commitment to someone or something.

  3. I will stop blaming others for my children's poor choices.

Parents and guardians, keeping your children safe and nurturing them is hard work. Like the Mother doe, it requires you protect them from harm while preparing them to conquer it themselves. It requires you keep them within your sight while allowing them to venture out of it.

It is the wise parent or guardian who errs on the side of safety and nurturance rather than going with the flow or doing what is popular or easy. In all my years of teaching, I never had a parent say, "I wish I hadn't known so much." Tragically, words commonly shared were, "I had no idea this was happening."

Even though you may encounter resistance as your children mature and as you make changes in your parenting, when you care for them over time while remaining cautious about detaching from them too early and being mindful of their need for independence and autonomy, you send to them several messages:

- They matter.

- They are valuable.

- They are important.

Pilates Routine: Reviewing the Safety and Nurturance exercises, choose one area which needs your attention the most. Work on that area for at least three weeks or until it becomes second nature to you and your children. Then, add another area of concern. Go slowly. This is not a race. It is better to do one or two things well than trying to accomplish too much too fast.

Parents and guardians, you can do this. Remember, your children have already made you the most important person in their lives. They deserve no less from you.

Do your homework. Keep going and keep growing.

Suggested Activity: After making changes in how you are providing safety and nurturance for your children for several weeks, select a day and time and respond to the following prompts.

- What have you discovered, about your children and yourself?

- How do you currently feel about doing what is best for your children rather than what is easy or popular?

Self-Assessment and Pacing Guide

It is time once again to conduct an honest assessment of your progress. Take a few moments, read over the criteria, and determine if you are ready or not to move forward.

Green Light: I have continued with daily Warm Ups #1 and #2. In addition, I have successfully integrated healthy changes in each of the three areas of Workout #1 Being Present. In Workout #2 Protecting, I utilized the Safety Questions to implement Protecting Exercises #1 and #2 - Safety, and I continue to utilize them in making decisions around protecting my children. I have answered the Nurturance questions and identified areas of strength and weakness in Protecting Exercise #3 - Nurturance. I have targeted areas which need improvement and implemented at least three actions steps in each area for a minimum of three weeks. I feel confident in my progress. My children have given me positive feedback.

Move on to Workout #1.

Red Light: I have fallen short in meeting my commitments in the daily Warm Ups or Workout #1. I need to stop, go back, and recommit to them before moving on.

Although I have maintained my commitments to the daily Warm Ups and exercises in Workout #1, I haven't done anything or I've done very little on Workout #2. I'm ready now to recommit to Pilates Workout #2: Protecting Exercises #1 and #2 and Nurturance Exercise #3. I will utilize the Safety Questions for making decisions or for redo's. In Nurturance Exercise #3, I will identify one area which needs improvement and implement three or more action steps for twenty-one consecutive days before adding another area of concern. I realize this may take me months to do. I am committed for however long it takes.

You'll find Protecting Exercises #1, #2 - Safety, and Protecting Exercise #3 - Nurturance below.

Recall a recent decision and reflect upon your decision-making process.

Pilates Workout #2: Protecting Exercise #1 – Safety

1. How much did I know about this person, place, thing, activity, etc.? Did I do my research, conduct background checks, or consult with trusted knowledgeable sources? What did I learn?

2. Why did I agree to this? Why did I disagree?

3. How did this benefit my children? How did it not?

4. Did I commit to monitoring, supervising, or following-up with this person, place, or thing, etc.? Did I explore my children's degree of involvement and how they were being affected or impacted? If so, what did that commitment look like?

The second exercise stretched you a bit further. You were asked to apply the Safety Questions to a current decision or a redo.

Pilates Workout #2: Protecting Exercise #2 - Safety

1. Identify a current decision or a redo on a past decision regarding your children and their safety.

2. Utilizing the criteria in the Safety Questions, work through each of the questions as you process your decision.

3. Talk with your children about your decision. Explain how and why you came to your decision.

4. Listen to your children's concerns. Answer their questions. Make adjustments as needed and as you gather more information.

5. Keep communication open between your children and you. Let them know how much they matter.

Pilates Workout #2: Protecting Exercise #3 - Nurturance

Within each question, there are multiple questions. Where applicable answer "yes, no, or sometimes." Then provide at least two examples to support your answers on the remaining questions.

1. Do I watch over my children (with electronic monitoring and in face to face supervision)? Do I know where they are, what they are doing, and with whom – in their net neighborhood and their real one?

2. Did I start out strong in my commitment to nurturance when my children were young and have I sustained that commitment over time? If so, in what ways? If not, what areas do I need to improve?

3. Have I exposed my children prematurely or allowed unsupervised access too early to a person, place, thing, etc., without considering their safety? Have I adequately prepared them with the appropriate insights and tools to handle potential dangers and possible harm? What areas do I need to address?

4. While caring for my children over time, am I being mindful of their needs for independence and autonomy? Am I encouraging them to make decisions on their own(age appropriately), to take on responsibilities, and to experience failure as well as success?

After you have answered the Nurturance Questions and provided examples to support your findings, take a deep breath. Acknowledge both your strengths and weaknesses. Then, respond to the following questions.

- What is the most important area I need to work on?

    1. Write down one area of concern.

    2. Then, identify three action steps to address that area.

    3. Implement the actions steps for three weeks or until they are a part of your behavior before adding another.

Pilates Workout #3:
Am I Meeting My Children's Needs While Being An Effective Mentor and Model?

In our "Pilates For Parenting" workout program, the exercises have been intentionally placed in their order of importance. Therefore, as we continue to add another workout, make sure you are staying committed to the Warm Ups – I Matter and My Children Matter, Workout #1 – Being Present, and Workout #2 – Protecting. Remember, they are foundational. Let's continue to flex and fortify our parent-child relationship.

Let's move on the Pilates Workout #3 – Providing and Guiding

Parenting books are filled with the latest suggestions on how to provide for children and how to fulfill your roles in guiding them. Families should absolutely tailor recommendations according to their values, belief systems, and traditional or cultural practices. For the purposes of "Pilates For Parenting," we will define Providing and Guiding in the following way:

Meeting my children's needs while being an effective mentor and model.

Read again, aloud.

Meeting my children's needs while being an effective mentor and model.

Although this concept may seem simplistic at first, its application carries with it enormous responsibility and self-accountability. First, as you strive to meet your children's needs, it is important to differentiate between needs and wants. Needs are requirements necessary for the promotion of wellbeing; whereas wants are defined as having the desire to possess or do something which may or may not enhance our wellbeing. As parents and guardians, it is critical you keep a pulse on what is needed and what is wanted, especially as our access and exposure to as well as consumption of anything has increased exponentially.

For example, through digital communication and interaction, we are becoming increasingly conditioned to feeding our wants in extremely efficient and timely ways. We see a pair of shoes we want. With one-click ordering, we can get it the same day or the next. A new video game is released. With online ordering at our fingertips, it's ours immediately. We want to check in with a friend so we send a text, expecting a quick reply. However, with this ease of self-gratification there can be consequences. When children are raised in environments of over-indulgence and given rewards without accomplishment, they often develop characteristics of entitlement and learned helplessness. Therefore, it is the responsibility of parents and guardians to acknowledge and meet your children's needs, not their wants.

Secondly, but as importantly, as parents and guardians work hard to meet their children's needs, they must also serve as mentors and models for them. In other words, you cannot say one thing, and do another, and then expect them to respect your roles as parents and guardians. In order to be an effective mentor and model, you must walk your talk and practice what you preach. If you want your children to embrace the values, beliefs, and standards you hold as important for healthy living, you must live by example and be accountable for it.

Let's get started with the concept of Providing as we examine two areas of attention.

- Physiological needs

- Psychological needs

Physiological Needs

Children's basic physiological needs such as food, shelter, and clothing are extremely important for their healthy development. If children are deprived of these basic needs, other areas of growth are jeopardized and can result in delayed development or other adverse effects.

On the other end of the spectrum, because many populations live in material-driven cultures, it is easy for parents to succumb to the pressures of staying up with the latest fads or competing with one another. Children want to fit in with their peers and most parents don't want their children to do without.

When speaking to audiences about achieving a healthy balance with technology in their lives, I'm often asked two questions. First, how old should my children be before I give them a smart phone? Secondly, how many hours a day is healthy for my children to be on their screens? In answering their questions, I always refer to years of research and publications from experts to support recommended guidelines. Parents and guardians are shocked to hear how it is best to delay turning over a smart phone to children twelve and under. And when I begin to share the guidelines from the American Academy of Pediatrics around the limited number of hours all children should be exposed to screens, there is usually a huge sigh of disbelief followed by resistance. Why? Because most parents and guardians don't want their children to do without or to be different than their friends.

However, as we have discussed, there are valuable lessons to be learned around what is needed and what is wanted. It's up to parents to make those distinctions and discuss the differences between them with their children. In addition, it is the responsibility of parents to become informed about the health consequences of any "want" and to supply their children with healthy alternatives while thoroughly explaining their rationale.

A couple of years ago, I attended a forum sponsored by the Family Online Safety Institute (FOSI). Tiffany, who was one of the keynote speakers and an award-winning short documentary filmmaker, described how she and her husband delayed turning over a smart phone to their adolescent and teen daughters until each turned fifteen, and they greatly limited their access to social net-working sites. Tiffany detailed how many other parents couldn't understand why they would deprive their daughters of having smart phones, and she disclosed how her older daughter was often teased by classmates. However, Tiffany and her husband, who worked in the field of robotics, understood the health consequences and stuck by their decisions. More importantly, Tiffany shared how their teen daughter thanked both parents for delaying her access after witnessing many of her friends struggle with personal, relational, and social issues regarding technology usage.

Providing the basic needs of children is essential for optimizing their healthy development and long-term wellbeing. Let's insure our parenting reflects that.

Psychological Meeds

Along with meeting your children's physiological needs, parents and guardians are charged with caring for their psychological wellbeing. This means you are responsible for the promotion of their healthy mental and emotional development. Although there are numerous areas which could be discussed, for the purposes of "Pilates For Parenting," we are going to focus on three interdependent components: unconditional love, belonging, and acceptance.

Unconditional Love

Children need unconditional love. Although this may sound profoundly obvious, it deserves our attention. Love means many different things to many different people. Thus, when we think about love for our children, it is comprised of deeply-felt emotions such as affection, attachment, caring, devotion, protection, and unconditional regard. As we implement "Pilates For Parenting," it is not enough to feel these emotions, but it is how these emotions are acted upon which will promote the healthy development of your children.

First, as children grow and mature they move through a series of developmental stages. At each stage, how parents and guardians respond to their children's needs greatly impacts their psychological and social wellbeing. For example, hearing their newborns' cries, parents and guardians respond by meeting their infant's needs for food, clothing, comfort, and cleanliness. Although most parents respond instinctively to their babies, when these basic needs are met in timely and consistent ways, trust – the first psychosocial developmental stage—begins to form with their parents and in their attachment to them.

Therefore, in order for your children to reach their healthy emotional potential, it is critical to be aware of their stages of development and become informed of the psychological and social needs within each stage. Providing unconditional love means deliberately funneling your emotions into actions to promote positive healthy outcomes. More information on the stages of development is provided in Appendix C: Erik Erikson's Stages of Psychosocial Development.

Secondly, children need unconditional love to be communicated and demonstrated. Many parents and guardians express their love for their children through verbal and written communications. This is a good start. However, "Pilates For Parenting" stretches the concept further. Parents and guardians must also support their expressions of love through their actions. As we thoroughly discussed in Workout #1 – Being Present, you show your children you love them by being available, being child-focused, and being a safe harbor. When your expressions of love are supported by and are congruent with your actions, children feel secure in their parents' love for them.

Lastly, children need to feel they are lovable. In other words, how parents and guardians approach their parenting contributes greatly to a child's sense of lovability. Although there are dozens of theories on parenting and hundreds of books on different approaches, for our series "Pilates For Parenting," we will break it down into three concise categories.

1. **Authoritarian parenting:** Authoritarian parenting lends itself to strict obedience, punitive measures, and rigid rules. Parents and guardians hold all power and control, with children having little or no voice. Authoritarian parenting creates confusion, fear, shame, and insecurity within children as they attempt to reconcile being loved within harsh and restrictive environments.

2. **Permissive parenting:** Overly permissive and neglectful approaches to parenting are also not conducive to instilling a sense of being loved within children. Although some children who are given free reign or who are left to fend for themselves may develop a premature sense of autonomy or independence, most children internalize their lack of parenting as not being worthy enough or not mattering enough to love.

3. **Authoritative parenting:** Authoritative parenting is in alignment with the connotations of unconditional love. Parenting is respectful, truthful, dependable, and flexible. Authoritative parenting blends empathy, compassion, and understanding into their parenting approach. This, in turn, cultivates an innate trust in the parent-child relationship, strengthens a healthy attachment, and instills a strong sense of lovability and of being enough within our children.

Parents and guardians, this is a lot to take in. For now, reflect upon these three approaches to parenting. In the Cool Down, you will be given the opportunity to assess and address your current style of parenting and to determine the kind of parent you want to be.

Parents and guardians, children need your unconditional love. They need it to be purposeful as you attach to them, and they need your love to be intentional as they navigate the stages of development. It is also important you not only express your love but you show it.

It is the extraordinary parent or guardian whose parenting approaches and behaviors embody the characteristics of unconditional love.

Belonging

Children need a sense of belonging. Belonging means to feel a part of a meaningful entity or unit. Having a strong sense of belonging within a family tethers children to their sense of worth and esteem while nourishing their confidence. Although their individual characters and personalities must be recognized, children who feel their unique and special being is an important piece of a whole tend to have greater feelings of self-efficacy. When children are neglected or when siblings are favored, they blame themselves and internalize it as self-deficiency.

Another important aspect of belonging for children is feeling they have a voice in their families. A sense of belonging is strengthened when children feel safe to express themselves and when their contributions are valued. When children are raised in environments which are overly critical of their words and behaviors, it is damaging to their self-image and their capacity to form healthy attachments.

A friend of mine, Sasha, recently shared an important story with me regarding belonging and the important of voice. After experiencing several serious struggles with her teenage daughter, Chloe, Sasha and her husband sought out family counseling. One of the most important findings in therapy was because Chloe was adopted by Sasha and her husband and her little brother was their biological child, Chloe did not feel as though she belonged in the family. And, Chloe did not want to express those feelings, thinking she may hurt others. In therapy, all family members learned how to express themselves and how each voice was valuable. After therapy concluded, Sasha shared how her family continued to have family meetings where everyone's voice was heard, bringing them all closer together.

Children need to feel their being holds a special place within the family. It is an exceptional family where their children's voices are encouraged and nurtured within the safety of the family unit.

Acceptance

Children need acceptance. At first, acceptance may seem to be the same as belonging. However, it is different. Children need to be celebrated for who they are. Each child is unique. Each child has her own personality, talents, quirks, creativity, strengths, and weaknesses. Each child must be celebrated for who she is and what she brings to the world. Each deserves the respect and the unconditional positive regard from her parent/s or guardians. A lack of acceptance causes children to feel ashamed of who they are. They often question their reason for being.

I don't have too many regrets as a parent, but there is one lesson which I wish I learned a little earlier than I did. When I had a daughter, I was thrilled. I loved dressing her up, braiding her long thick hair, and enrolling her in dance class. I have to say, she was a good sport. However, by about age five, I noticed she would rather wear a baseball cap, dig in the dirt, and ride her little tricycle. After a disastrous dance recital followed by a teary-eyed little girl who didn't like being dressed up like Dorothy in the Wizard of Oz, I finally saw the light. I stopped trying to make her into the dainty princess I thought she should be, and I started accepting and celebrating her for the incredibly strong, independent, and outgoing spirit she was...and still is!

It is the responsibility of parents and guardians to create an environment of acceptance within the family. It is the remarkable family who celebrates the uniqueness of each individual child.

As we think about meeting the psychological needs of our children and the lasting impact on their lives, this is important.

Providing unconditional love, belonging, and acceptance cultivates a deep sense of worth and value within a child. Not doing so creates significant disequilibrium around their sense of self and an inability to form healthy attachments as they grow and mature.

Read it again, slowly and aloud.

Providing unconditional love, belonging, and acceptance cultivates a deep sense of worth and value within a child. Not doing so creates significant disequilibrium around their sense of self and an inability to form healthy attachments as they grow and mature.

Take a deep breath and move on with "Providing Exercise #1"

Parents and guardians, while reflecting on the above concepts, assess how you are providing for your children's physiological and psychological needs. Take as much time as you need responding to these questions. Take out your journal or other writing materials.

Pilates Workout #3: Providing Exercise #1 – Physiological and Psychological Needs

Some questions contain multiple questions. Where applicable, answer "yes, no, or sometimes." Then, provide at least two examples to support your answers on the remaining questions.

1. Am I providing three basic essentials: food, shelter, and clothing? For example:

    *   Yes, I am providing food, shelter, and clothing.

        1. I make sure my children have nutritious food and enough food.

        2. My children don't have a lot of clothes, but what they do have is clean, in good repair, and comfortable.

2. Am I meeting their physiological needs or am I succumbing to their wants? Am I explaining the differences to them? For example:

- Sometimes I do give in to them when I know it is not a good idea.

    1. My son wants more video games and I buy them for him.

    2. I haven't explained the differences. We usually just argue about it.

3. As my children grow, am I aware of their stages of development and is my love for them intentional and purposeful? Am I expressing my love, both in my words and my actions? Is how I parent consistent with my messages of love so that my children feel lovable? For example:

    - No, I am not aware of the stages of development and how I love them may impact those stages.

        1. I've read a few parenting books, but they did not talk about the developmental stages.

        2. Sometimes I feel overly-protective of my children and I am wondering if that is a good thing.

    - Yes, I show and express my love.

        1. I tell my children that I love them every day.

        2. After working on the exercises in Workout #1 Being Present, I am showing my love by following through on my commitments to them.

    - Sometimes my parenting is consistent with my messages of love.

        1. Although I want my older children to be more independent, I am too screen-attached to them. I'm always texting them and making their decisions for them.

        2. Sometimes, when I'm tired and stressed, I yell at my children. I've seen them cry.

4. Am I providing a sense of belonging for my children so they feel connected to the family unit? Do my children feel safe to express themselves? For example:

    - Sometimes I think our family is really disconnected.

        1. We are usually on our technology not paying attention to one another.

        2. Much of the time at home, my children are alone in their bedrooms on their technology.

    - Yes and no.

        1. I think my children feel connected to me.

        2. I don't think my step-children feel like a part of our family.

- Sometimes my children feel safe to express themselves.

    1. We don't talk a lot as a family. When we do, I think they feel safe.

    2. I don't always agree with my teenage daughter. I get mad at her and she shuts down. I don't think she feels her voice matters.

5. Do I accept my children for who they are or am I critical, judgmental, or do I find fault with them? Have I asked them if they feel accepted by me or if they feel lovable? Have I asked them if they feel like "they are enough?" For example:

    - Yes, I accept my children for who they are.

        1. Each of my children is very unique. They have different talents and interests and I support them fully.

        2. Because I was criticized as a child, I do not judge or criticize my children.

    - No, I have never thought to ask them if my children feel accepted, lovable, or enough.

        1. I assumed my children feel accepted by me.

        2. Now, I wonder how they will answer.

After you have answered the Providing Questions and given examples to support your findings, take a deep breath. Acknowledge both your strengths and weaknesses. Then, respond to the following:

- What is the most important area I need to work on?

    1. Write down one area of concern.

    2. Then, identify three action steps to address that area.

    3. Implement the action steps for three weeks or until they are a part of your behavior before adding another. For example:

- Area of concern: Sometimes I think our family is really disconnected.

    1. We are going to keep and use all our technology in one room of the house.

    2. We are going to shut down and put all our technology away before we go to bed.

    3. We are going to put our technology away at dinner and talk to one another.

Parents and guardians, this workout is extremely important. So, take your time. You may also find as you address one area of concern, you might also be able to address another. Again, this is the beauty of Pilates. As we target one area, we strengthen a related area.

When you are ready, move on to our second Pilates practice—*Guiding*. We will explore two areas:

- Mentoring

- Modeling

Mentoring

Mentoring is a common term which we typically associate with an experienced individual who is training a novice or less knowledgeable person in a specific field or task. For the purposes of "Pilates For Parenting," we are going to define mentoring as the following:

Teaching and guiding my children as they move through their developmental stages so they will be better prepared to navigate their world confidently.

Let's read again, aloud.

Teaching and guiding my children as they move through their developmental stages so they will be better prepared to navigate their world confidently.

First, in order to be an effective mentor, you must be a teacher who is keenly self-aware. You must take into consideration how your childhood histories and background experiences are influencing or impacting your mentoring.

For example, parents and guardians who grew up feeling they fell short of a goal or did not reach their full potential often try to compensate for or to fill their unmet needs through their children. This can place extraordinary pressure on children as they try to please their parents and earn their love. It is absolutely beneficial to children's development when parents provide their children with diverse athletic opportunities, artistic avenues, and academic endeavors. However, this does not mean you should expect children to follow in your footsteps or they must embrace the interests you engaged in as children. Effective mentoring means you teach your children by sharing both the successes and failures you experienced in following your dreams while making room for them discover their passions.

Secondly, being an effective mentor means you guide your children as you prepare them to be autonomous and independent. In "Workout #1 – Being Present", we discussed the importance of parents being a safe harbor for their children. Mentoring adds another dimension to this metaphor. Thus, as you mentor, children need to know you will provide a consistent compass for them to tether their decision-making and to assist in their course of action. At the same time, whether your children are successful or not, constructive mentoring means they should be given leeway to discover their purpose and uncover their passions even as they struggle through developmental challenges and changes.

In conversations with my husband about mentoring, Dan always references his dad. Starting at a young age, Dan's father took Dan everywhere with him performing various jobs. Dan worked alongside his dad learning carpentry skills such as building lath houses to provide shade structures for plants. At a local nursery, Dan's dad taught him how to care for plants and instructed him on basic landscaping skills. At age twelve, Dan's father owned a gas station. Until his graduation from high school, Dan worked with his dad, after school and on weekends preforming a multitude of jobs including servicing and repairing cars. However, throughout the years of mentoring in his father's areas of expertise, Dan's dad always encouraged Dan to do well in school, and he strongly supported Dan's passion to pursue an advanced degree in education. To this day, Dan credits his father for shaping his work ethic while molding his moral compass.

While effective mentoring requires parents and guardians to instruct and guide their children, it is also important to be available and present to talk through issues, problem solve, and assist children in making responsible informed decisions. Of course, younger children require more direction and guidance. In addition, effective mentoring means tailoring your approach to the individual needs and personality of each child. Most importantly, you must be willing to ask your children for their feedback, remaining open and receptive to their thoughts and feelings and making adjustments where needed.

Although there are times where is it beneficial for children to experience the consequences of their behaviors or choices and to learn from them, when children are left adrift to figure it out for themselves, without informed guidance, the consequences can be dangerous and at times deeply damaging.

It is the strongly aware parent or guardian who provides a consistent compass for their children while allowing them to take the wheel as they learn to chart their course.

Modeling

Parents and guardians have heard this word a lot. However, its importance cannot be emphasized enough. In traditional terms, modeling is defined as showing our children how to do something or demonstrating the desired behavior through the process of imitation. For our purposes in "Pilates For Parenting," we will define it as the following:

Modeling means parenting by example.

Read slowly again. Absorb the impact of its significance.

Modeling means parenting by example.

This is important. Modeling does not mean you have to be perfect. It means you need to be consistent with and conscious of your behaviors as you establish expectations and norms for your children. If you do not practice what you preach or if you do not model the behaviors you hope to instill in your children, they will learn that too.

In "Workout # 3 Providing and Guiding," I talked about Tiffany and her husband and their decision to delay giving smart phones to their teen and adolescent daughters until they reached age fifteen. At the same conference, Tiffany also shared how everyone in her family took part in creating their Family Media Plan, which consisted not only of designated times for tech usage but also of carefully crafted opportunities for face to face time. One example she described still remains with me and I share it often with audiences.

Because Tiffany and her family are Jewish, for over eight years they have been practicing "Tech Shabbat"! From Friday at sundown until Saturday at sundown, all (and I mean all) technology is turned off and put away. Tiffany and her family plan out various activities, giving everyone a voice in the decisions: biking, hiking, going to a museum, playing board games, etc. Tiffany said how over the years, there have been many times where her family decided to extend the tech-free time, realizing how much they enjoyed really connecting with one another. At the end of her presentation, Tiffany shared this important piece. At first, Tiffany and her husband were worried they may be missing out on important work issues or other communications. However, they quickly realized if they wanted to demonstrate the importance of honoring their commitment to spending quality time with one another, they too must model the behaviors.

This is important.

What you say matters. What you do matters more.

Read it again, aloud.

What you say matters. What you do matters more.

Your children are observing and learning from you. They can spot a hypocrite a mile away. Parenting by example will have a lasting impact on your children.

It is the wise parent or guardian who understands this. It is the model parent who puts it to work.

Let's continue.

Pilates Workout #3: Guiding Exercise #1 – Mentoring and Modeling

Spend time reflecting on the following questions. Take your time. Remember, we don't have to change everything at once. However, when it comes to mentoring and modeling, it is important to be brutally honest with ourselves. Therefore, carve out an hour or so when you have some alone, quiet time. Take out your journal or other writing materials. Take a deep breath. Remember, as you stretch yourself, you strengthen the parent-child relationship.

Within each question, there are multiple questions. Where applicable, answer "yes, no, or sometimes." Then, provide at least two examples to support your answers.

1. Do I expect my children to be like me or follow my dreams or do I cultivate their unique characters and support their passions? Am I checking in with them to see how they feel? For example:

   - I'm a little upset by the question. I'm feeling guilty.

     1. I introduced sports to my children because I loved sports.

     2. They seem to love it and have never complained.

   - No, I haven't checked in with them.

      1. I need to talk to them.

      2. My daughter asked about playing a musical instrument and I sort of brushed it off.

2. As my children grow and develop, am I a reliable compass or are they trying to figure it out by themselves? Have I asked for their feedback?

- Yes, I believe I am a reliable compass.

      1. Whenever they have a problem, we discuss and solve it together.

      2. When a decision needs to be made, I help them look at the pros and cons to all sides.

- Sometimes I ask for their feedback.

      1. I will commit to ask for their feedback.

      2. I will set a time on a weekly basis to do so.

3. Am I modeling the kinds of behaviors and attitudes I want to instill in my children or do I have the same expectations for myself that I have for my children? Am I asking my family for their feedback?

    For example:

- Sometimes I model the behaviors and want to instill in my children.

      1. I need to put my phone away when I come home if I want them to cut back on using theirs.

      2. I want them to pay attention when I am speaking to them, but I don't always pay attention to them.

- No, I have not asked my family for their feedback.

      1. I don't know how they feel.

      2. I don't know if I set a good example.

4. When I see my children misbehaving or mistreating someone or something, have I asked them where they learned the behavior? Am I willing to listen to their responses? How will I respond?

- No, I have not asked my children where they learned the behavior.

      1. I usually just get upset with them.

      2. I usually blame someone else.

- Yes, I will ask them and I am willing to listen to their responses.

      1. We will talk about it.

2. If my children learned it from me, I will learn from my mistakes and tell them.

After you have answered the Guiding Questions and given support for your findings, take a deep breath. Acknowledge your strengths and weaknesses. Then, respond to the following:

- What is the most important area I need to work on?

  1. Write down one area of concern.

  2. Then, identify three action steps to address that area.

  3. Implement the action steps for three weeks or until they are a part of your behavior before adding another. For example:

- Area of concern: I'm a little upset and worried that I have expected my children to like what I like and follow in my footsteps.

  1. I'm going to have an honest talk with them.

  2. I'm going to ask them if there is anything else they would rather be doing or exploring.

  3. I will support them in their choices.

This is a lot to digest. Although Mentoring and Modeling, along with Meeting My Children's Needs, are placed last in our exercise routine, they are extremely important. Parents and guardians, you are your children's first attachments and teachers. And whether you realize it or not, as they grow and develop, you still remain the most influential persons in their lives.

Pilates Routine: The Pilates principles of Providing and Guiding are not easy to assess and address. And, they require a commitment to implementing them on a daily basis. Again, go slowly. Take your time. Choose one area to work on for at least three weeks or until it feels a natural part of your routine. Add another area when you feel ready.

Just as is true with any exercise regimen, the more you work out and the more you integrate these practices into your routine, they will take hold of you, providing and guiding you in your parenting journey.

Keep stretching yourself and strengthening your family.

Suggested Activity: After making a few shifts in your providing of your children's needs (unconditional love, belonging, and acceptance) and in guiding them (mentoring and modeling), select a day and time to respond to the following prompts.

- What am I learning about myself as a provider of my children's needs?

- What am I learning about my children?

- What areas have I improved upon as a mentor and model? Which is more difficult for me? How will I continue to stretch myself?

Self-Assessment and Pacing Guide

It is time once again to conduct an honest assessment of your progress. Take a few moments, read over the criteria, and determine if you are ready or not to move forward.

Green Light: I have continued with daily Warm Ups #1 and #2. In addition, I have successfully integrated healthy changes in each of the three areas of Workout #1 Being Present and in both areas of Workout #2 – Protecting. In Workout #3, I have addressed the questions in Providing Exercise #1 and identified areas of strength and weakness in meeting my children's physiological and psychological needs. I have targeted one area at a time which needed improvement and implemented three actions steps for a minimum of three weeks.

I moved on to Guiding Exercise #2, responded to the questions on mentoring and modeling and identified areas of concern. I have targeted areas which need improvement and implemented at least three actions steps in each area for a minimum of three weeks. I feel confident in my progress. My children have given me positive feedback.

Move on to Cool Down.

Red Light: I have fallen short in meeting my commitments in the daily Warm Ups, Workout #1 or Workout #2. I need to stop, go back, and recommit to them before moving on.

I have maintained my commitments to the daily Warm Ups, and to the exercises in Workouts #1 and #2; however, I haven't done anything or I've done very little on Workout #3. I'm ready now to recommit to Pilates Workout #3: Providing Exercises #1 and Guiding Exercise #2. I will utilize the Providing Questions for assessing how well I am meeting my children's physiological and psychological needs and target one area of concern at a time. I will implement actions steps for three weeks before adding another area. In Guiding Exercise #2, I will respond to the questions on mentoring and modeling. I will identify one area which needs improvement and implement three or more action steps for twenty-one consecutive days before adding another area of concern. I realize this may take me months to do. I am committed for however long it takes.

You'll find Providing Exercise #1 and Guiding Exercise #2 on the following pages.

Pilates Workout #3:
Providing Exercise #1 – Physiological and Psychological Needs

1. Am I providing three basic essentials: food, shelter, and clothing?

2. Am I meeting their physiological needs or am I succumbing to their wants? Am I explaining the differences to them?

3. As my children grow, am I aware of their stages of development and is my love for them intentional and purposeful? Am I expressing my love, both in my words and my actions? Is how I parent consistent with my messages of love so that my children feel lovable?

4. Am I providing a sense of belonging for my children so they fell connected to the family unit? Do my children feel safe to express themselves?

5. Do I accept my children for who they are or am I critical, judgmental, or do I find fault with them? Have I asked them if they feel accepted by me or have I asked if they feel like "they are enough?"

After you answered the Providing Questions and gave examples to support your findings, you were also encouraged to acknowledge both your strengths and weaknesses. Then, you were asked to respond to the following:

- What is the most important area I need to work on?

    1. Write down one area of concern.

    2. Then, identify three action steps to address that area.

    3. Implement the action steps for three weeks or until they are a part of your behavior before adding another.

Pilates Workout #3:
Guiding Exercise #1 – Mentoring and Modeling

1. Do I expect my children to be like me or follow my dreams or do I cultivate their unique characteristics and support their passions? Am I checking in with them to see how they feel?

2. As my children grow and develop, am I a reliable compass or are they trying to figure it out for themselves? Have I asked for their feedback?

3. Am I modeling the kinds of behaviors and attitudes I want to instill in my children or do I have the same expectations for myself that I have for my children? Am I asking my family for their feedback?

4. When I see my children misbehaving or mistreating someone or something, have I asked them to share where they learned the behavior? Am I willing to listen to their responses? How will I respond?

After you answered the Guiding Questions and gave support for your findings, you were encouraged to acknowledge your strengths and weaknesses. Then, you were asked to respond to the following:

*   What is the most important area I need to work on?

    1. Write down one area of concern.

    2. Then, identify three action steps to address that area.

    3. Implement the action steps for three weeks or until they are a part of your behavior before adding another.

Pilates Cool Down. Not Perfection But Purposeful

As we begin our Cool Down, let's keep in mind when parents and guardians provide for children's physical and psychological needs and when they guide their paths, children feel lovable, worthy, and valuable.

Let's continue to show them they matter as we fine-tune and fortify our parenting.

You have had quite a workout in "Pilates For Parenting!" The Warm Ups and Workouts are designed to introduce you to a set of principles and equip you with a set of practices to stretch and strengthen your parenting. These concepts and exercises are cultivating a deeper sense of awareness around their importance in raising your children and their impact on them.

While the Warm Ups and the Workouts target the core of "Pilates For Parenting," the Cool Down allows you to personalize your style of parenting. Why is that important? Each of you brings to your Pilates experience your past and your life messages about parent-child relationships. In addition, each of you is affected by diverse social, cultural, and economic forces. Therefore, it is important to take stock of both positive and negative influences in your lives and to integrate healthy practices within each of them which will grow and deepen the parent-child relationship.

As you think about everything you have learned, it is important to remember this truth.

I don't need to be perfect in my parenting. I need to be purposeful.

Repeat, slowly and aloud.

I don't need to be perfect in my parenting. I need to be purposeful.

Purposeful in a key word. It is an empowering word. For your children, it may be life-changing.

Being purposeful means parenting with intention and deliberate forethought. Being purposeful means knowing the answer to this question:

What kind of parent do I want to be?

Breathe in slowly. Breathe out slowly. Repeat.

What kind of parent do I want to be?

Let's continue.

Pilates Cool Down: Exercise #1 -
What Kind Of Parent Do I Want To Be?

The Cool Down Questions are extremely important. Do not rush this. Take as much time as you need. Answer one or two. Set it aside. Come back and work on the questions again. When reflecting on how you were parented, you may find some of these questions elicit painful memories. There may be other recollections which put a smile on your face. Each of you is unique. Honor your truths and learn from them. The more you put into this, the more you will gain from it.

Find a quiet time, alone. Take out your journal or other writing material. Get comfortable.

Answer each of the following questions. Write down at least three examples and explanations to support your responses.

1. Think about how you were parented. What worked for you? Why? What didn't? Why?

2. What beliefs, practices, or approaches are you replicating from your childhood? Are they healthy? Why or why not?

3. Are you over-compensating for what was unhealthy in your childhood? Explain and give examples. What will you commit to work on and let go of?

4. What positives behaviors do you see in how others parent? Provide examples and identify positives practices you will commit to implementing.

5. What other resources, belief systems, values, or foundational principles guide you in your parenting? Which help you to be the kind of parent you want to be? Why?

After you have finished answering the questions above, read over your responses and reflect upon them. Again, take as much time as you need. Take out your journal or other writing materials. Respond to the following prompts.

1. What are you learning today that you didn't know yesterday which will help you to be the kind of parent or guardian you want to be?

2. What action steps or behaviors will you implement today to become the parent or guardian you want to be?

Pilates Routine: Revisit Cool Down Exercise #1 often. As you go through struggles and successes with your children, it is helpful to learn from your past and glean from positive experiences. As additional healthy influences and sources become available, remain open and intentional about blending them into your daily mindset and routine. You never stop growing in your parenting.

As we prepare to conclude our time together, I'd like to share a personal story which relates to the Cool Down.

My parents were very young when they married and not equipped to handle the responsibilities. In addition, both parents were alcoholics, raising my three sisters and me in an environment which was riddled with criticism, harshness, and at times, chaos. In other words, our home was not stable, it was not child-focused, and it was not a safe harbor. At eleven years old I made two promises to myself.

First, even though at my young age I didn't have the vocabulary to describe my home environment or an understanding of addiction, I promised myself I would not repeat it. Secondly, I promised myself if I ever had the privilege of becoming a mother, I would parent differently than what I was experiencing. Although I have made poor decisions throughout my life and have endured hardship, I learned from those experiences and I embraced a recovering journey at an early age. Most importantly, I kept those two promises.

I have not been a perfect parent, but I have been a purposeful one. I took stock of what my childhood was like and how it impacted me. As I prepared to become a mother, I assessed and addressed the questions in "What Kind of Parent Do I Want To Be? And then, each and every step of the way, I intentionally chose to parent embracing the principles and practices I share with you: I Matter and My Children Matter; Being Present; Protecting; Providing and Guiding: Mentoring and Modeling; and Cool Down.

In addition, as I traveled my parenting journey, I reached out for healthy guidance and encouragement. It is my privilege to support you in yours.

As you continue to Stretch Yourself and Strengthen Your Family, take a deep breath. *Relax. Cool Down.*

And then, each and every day, begin anew. Recommit yourself again.

Remember.

I don't need to be perfect. I need to be purposeful.

Self-Assessment and Pacing Guide

Green Light: I continue to implement the daily Warm Ups and exercises in Workouts #1, #2, and #3. In addition, I have answered the questions in Cool Down Exercise #1 and the follow-up prompts. I am learning more about myself and how my past and other influences affect my parenting style. I am becoming the kind of parent I want to be and I am understanding why it is important. I do not need to be perfect. I commit to being a purposeful parent or guardian.

If I have not completed all aspects of the Warm Ups and Workouts, I commit to completing all aspects of "Pilates For Parenting" because I know...

I Matter To My Children and My Children Matter To Me

Why Can't You and I Have Mother – Son Date Night?

When my husband Dan and I married, my daughter Alexis, from my previous marriage, had just turned five. Dan had two teen children who spent the majority of the time with their mother. Shortly after our wedding, Dan approached Alexis about joining *Y Princess* (formerly called *Indian Y Princess*) – a father-daughter program which encourages fun, understanding, and companionship with one another and with other fathers and their daughters.

For the next several years, Alexis and Dan attended their monthly group, participating in and enjoying all kinds of adventurous activities. After moving to Southern California, Dan and Alexis found their new group not to be as organized or meaningful. With our work schedules changing as well, Dan proposed a weekly Father-Daughter date night to Alexis. She excitedly agreed.

During her third grade year, Alexis would wait patiently for Dan to come home for their date night. To make it more special, Alexis was given the freedom to choose what they would do or where they would go: bowling, playing video games, pool, or miniature golf; going out to dinner or to a movie; or whatever else she chose, within reason. Alexis loved her date night, as did Dan. He never disappointed her. He always made it home from work. He always kept his commitment.

Several months into the year, my step-son came to live with us. He was in high school and had not lived with us before. Needless to say, things were quite rocky as our family was trying to acclimate to an entirely new dynamic. Slowly and after some challenging situations and conversations, my relationship with my step-son started to improve. One night after Alexis and Dan left for their date night, my step-son and I sat at the dining room table eating our dinner.

Suddenly, he looked up at me and asked, "Holli, why can't you and I have Mother-Son date night?"

Although I was pleasantly surprised, it caught me off guard. "Well... I don't know..." Still feeling a bit uncertain, I needed reassurance. "Are you sure? I mean, I would love it! I just didn't know if you would want to hang out with me?"

He smiled and said, "Yeah.... I would."

From that week on, my step-son and I enjoyed our Mother-Son date night. It changed everything, for the better.

It's never too late to show your children they matter. *Never.*

Appendix A - Family Media Plan

The American Academy of Pediatrics provides a template for tailoring your Family Media Plan (see Appendix B). Or, families can come together and have a say in creating their unique plan. It's fun and easy to do. Plus, there is a stronger likelihood of buy-in.

As you develop your Family Media Plan, it is important to include the following:

1. All family members

2. All types of screens (including video gaming)

3. All family members agree to and sign their plan (except those too young to do so)

4. Screen usage: plans take into account age differences of children and recommendations from experts

   - Age: 0 - 18 months: no exposure to screens

   - Age: 18 months - 2 years: brief, interactive screen time with adults

   - Age: 2 - 12 years: 2 hours per day; interactive screen time with adults is recommended

   - Age: 13 - 18 years: 2 hours per day with negotiated responsible use

5. Plans may be renegotiated as needs, challenges, and issues surface

6. Placement of screens and designated screen-free times

   - All screens kept in one room at home

   - No screens during meal times

   - No screens allowed in bedrooms, ever

   - No screen exposure two hours before bedtime

7. Monitoring and supervising measures

   - Specific times are established for parents and guardians to check their children's social media accounts, texts, and other electronic communications

   - Random checks are also strongly recommended

- Parents and guardians discuss with their children the use of safety apps and other protective measures and delineate them in the Family Media Plan

8. Good digital citizenship expectations

- Families discuss and delineate acceptable online behaviors

- Parents and guardians discuss with children and delineate consequences for unacceptable online behaviors

- Children who receive any unsafe or unkind online messages agree to save it and share it with their parents and guardians

9. Social media guidelines

- Age 13 is the requirement for being on social media

- Limit: one or two accounts with approval of parents and guardians

10. Responsibility for screens

- Parents and guardians discuss with children and delineate appropriate use of each device (how it is to be used, when, and with whom)

- Parents and guardians discuss with children responsibilities of ownership (such as costs, damage to screens, etc.) and delineate accountability measures for them

Sample: Family Media Plan

Jones Family Media Plan

We, the Jones Family, want to have a healthy and safe relationship with our technology. We agree to the following:

1. **Placement of screens and designated screen-free times:**

    -   All screens will be kept and used in our family room (den)

    -   No screens in the bedrooms, including mom and dad

    -   No screens at meal times, including eating out

    -   No screens two hours before bedtime

    -   No screen usage in the car, truck, etc., except on long trips

2. **Screen Usage:** We all use our screens way too much. Aside from use at school or work, our current daily goals the following:

    -   Dad: one hour at home

    -   Mom: one hour at home

    -   Jason (age 16): two hours at home

    -   Angela (age 12): one hour at home

    -   Ricky (age 6): one hour with mom or dad

    -   We will watch TV together. No more than two hours per day

    -   We will replace screen time with playing games, reading books, and we will plan other activities, especially on the weekends

    -   Except for taking a few photos, we will not take out our screens when we are going other places, playing games, or participating in activities

3. **Monitoring, supervising, and good digital citizenship:**

    -   Jason has a smartphone. Jason is being responsible. Jason agrees to save and report any unsafe behavior to mom and dad. Jason agrees to sit down once a week to share his "net neighborhood" with Mom or Dad.

    -   Angela has a smartphone. Because there has been a lot of drama with friends, for the next two weeks Angela agrees to use her phone for texting only Mom, Dad, Jason, or other family members. Mom and Dad will check her phone weekly. Angela agrees to stay off social networking for one month.

    -   Little Ricky: Ricky plays a lot of video games. He will play one hour a day.

We, the Jones family, agree to come together each Sunday and talk about how our Family Media Plan is working. We agree to make adjustments as needed.

Mom_____   Dad _____

Jason_____   Angela _____

Ricky _____

Appendix B – Resources

1) **Academy of Pediatrics** www.healthychildren.org
   The American Academy of Pediatrics is your go-to website for a wealth of information including the following:

   - Template for a personalized Family Media Use Plan

   - Recommendations for media usage

   - Research-based articles on relevant health issues, disorders, and diseases as well as recommendations for intervention and treatment

2) **Cam Adair of "Game Quitters"** http://gamequitters.com
   Cam Adair is an incredible resource for anyone in the family struggling with gaming dependence or addiction. His website is friendly. Being a former game addict, Cam comes from a place of compassion and accountability. Some of his resources include the following:

   - Respawn Guide For Gamers

   - Reclaim Guide For Loved Ones

   - Parent Support Group

3) **Screen Strong** – An Initiative Of Families Managing Media https://screenstrong.com
   The mission statement from this phenomenal organization is the following: Families Managing Media empowers parents to confidently develop a balanced digital media lifestyle. Focusing on the connection between brain development and media use, we provide proven solutions to reclaim kids and reconnect families in today's digital world.
   Resources include by are not limited to the following:

   - Audio Seminars

   - Books

   - Interviews with Moms

4) **Family Online Safety Institute** – How To Be A Good Digital Parent www.fosi.org

Part of their Mission Statement reads as follows: The Family Online Safety Institute is an international, non-profit organization which works to make the online world safe for kids and their families.

FOSI has been dedicated to the health and wellbeing of your children for over a decade. Aside from their work around Policy and Research and Individual Best Practices, FOSI has developed a Good Digital Parenting Program. Its highlights include the following:

- Free materials, downloads, slides, etc.

- Instructions on how to present the Good Digital Parenting Program to parents, schools, organizations

- Support and guidance

5) **Screenagers & Dr. Delaney Ruston** https://www.screenagersmovie.com

Dr. Delaney Ruston is a medical doctor and film-maker. She and her team launched "Screenagers" several years ago. It continues to be an international success. "Screenagers" opens up the conversation about the challenges and struggles of raising kids in the digital age. More importantly, Dr. Ruston addresses some of the serious concerns around screen dependence.

For details on how to screen this film with your school, community, place of worship, etc., contact their website.

Dr. Ruston and her team have also developed a phone usage policy for elementary and middle schools, "Away For The Day." Everything needed to join this movement and begin implementing a policy in your district or school can be found at www.awayfortheday.org.

6) **Wait Until 8th** www.waituntil8th.org

Wait Until 8th is a grassroots organization started by parents who are concerned about their children's early exposure to screens and the ensuing consequences. Their mission statement is clear and strong: We empower parents to say yes to waiting for the smartphone.

Everything you need to start your own chapter or parent group of Wait Until Eighth is available on their website.

Appendix C –
Erik Erikson's Stages of Psycho-Social Development

As we discussed in Workout #3, providing for children's psychological needs means you not only feel unconditional love for them, but you also act upon your love in very specific and intentional ways. Although most parents respond to their children's needs instinctively, it is important to become knowledgeable about their stages of psycho-social development. By doing so, parents and guardians can tailor how they parent their children and respond to their needs in order to promote healthy psychological and social development.

There are many theories of human development. Even though there are some limitations to Erik Erikson's theory of life-span development, his work has been highly regarded throughout the field of psychology. A few important factors with regards to Erikson's theory include the following:

- For each age grouping, the span of years is flexible with some overlap.

- Within each stage, there are two opposing developmental outcomes: positive and negative.

- It is the goal of each stage of development to acquire positive outcomes.

- If a child does not achieve positive outcomes within a developmental stage, he or she enters the next stage at a disadvantage.

- As children grow, at any time and with guidance, intervention, and support, they can return to a previous stage and renegotiate it with positive outcomes.

In addition, as a therapist, I have found when children are victims of adverse childhood experiences such as trauma (such as a death, divorce), abuse, or neglect of physical and psychological needs, this significantly impacts or interrupts their healthy psycho-social development. In other words, a child can be thriving but when traumatized at any given age, that child is unlikely to navigate that stage of development successfully. Furthermore, unless there is appropriate intervention, the child's development through the ensuing stages is most likely to be diminished or arrested. Because psychology is not an exact science, it is difficult to draw absolute conclusions for any child without considering all factors involved.

Let's take a look at the first five stages of psycho-social development and their desired outcomes. For our purposes, I have paraphrased Erikson's theory to make it Pilates-friendly.

Stage One (0 – 18 months): Mistrust vs. Basic Trust

From birth until about 18 months, children's needs are centered around their physical and psychological comfort. It is important parents and guardians tend to their needs for food, clothing, cleanliness, safety and shelter. It is critical parents and guardians bond with their infants through various forms of touch, facial expression, tone of voice, and social interaction. Most importantly, there must be consistency and continuity in their responses to meeting their children's needs.

Because babies are dependent entirely upon their parents and guardians to comfort them, when their needs are not met in timely and thorough ways or when they are neglected, infants become fearful and mistrusting of their environments. They often fail to thrive or form attachments to their caregivers.

- **Pilates Pointer:** When infants' physical and psychological needs are met in tender, thoughtful, and timely ways, they feel secure. They develop positive outcomes of trust and attachment.

Stage Two (18 months – 3 years): Shame and Doubt vs. Autonomy

We all joke about the terrible two's! And yet, this is such an important stage of development. As early as 18 months, children begin to assert their independence. They are discovering their behavior is their own and they have free will. Although toddlers still need their parents and guardians to fill their needs for comfort and safety, they are becoming aware of their autonomy, realizing they can do things on their own. While protecting them from harm, it is important parents and guardians allow their toddlers to explore, investigate, and try new things. It is critical for little ones to have the freedom to play, create, make a mess, and feel valued for their independent nature. Developing a strong sense of autonomy is a positive outcome at this stage of development.

Being overly-protective is an understandable response to this stage, but it promotes self-doubt as toddles are restrained from engaging or exploring. In addition, parents and guardians who punish children harshly for their independent nature or who constantly correct them create a core of anxiety and shame.

- **Pilates Pointer:** Allow your children the freedom to express their will and independent nature. Create safe environments for them to do so. Gently and lovingly redirect them when they venture into harm's way.

Stage Three (3 – 6 years): Guilt vs. Initiative

Pre-school children begin to encounter a widening social world. As they do so, they face new and challenging responsibilities. They are learning to take ownership of their bodies, to be accountable for their behaviors, and to take care of things which are important to them such as toys and pets. Children who are guided to take responsibility and encouraged in positive ways develop a strong sense of purpose and initiative. Whether there is successful completion of tasks or when children experience setbacks or failures, it is extremely important for parents and guardians to respond with compassion, guidance, and encouragement.

Not wanting your children to fail is a normal feeling for most parents. However, when children are not challenged by accepting responsibility for themselves and their behaviors, they internalize feelings of helplessness and inadequacy. As a result, children become less likely to initiate purposeful behavior. In addition, when parents and guardians respond to their children's behaviors with criticism or harsh correction, children become anxious and blame themselves. Feeling guilty for their lack of accomplishment, children are less like to take on responsibility.

- **Pilates Pointer:** Provide ample opportunities for your children to take on responsibilities, especially as their social world widens. Lovingly guide and support them. Reinforce their successes and reframe their setbacks as opportunities to learn.

Stage Four (6 – 12 years): Inferiority vs. Industry

As children move into middle and late childhood, they have a strong need to increase their knowledge and to master interests and skills. Because their enthusiasm is greatly enhanced during these developmental years, it is extremely important they are encouraged to explore their areas of interest. As children learn, create, practice or train, it is critical they begin to feel competent in their abilities, talents, and gifts. It is also during this stage of development where children begin to produce significant evidence of their competencies: recitals, performances, competitive sports, report cards, etc. Validating children as they pursue their passions and affirming their accomplishments will strengthen a sense of industry (competence).

Most parents and guardians want their children to be successful. This is natural. However, when parents or guardians set expectations too high or are overly critical of their children's level of achievement, children internalize this as self-deficiency or not being enough. They develop feelings of incompetence, inferiority, and shame. Also, as we discussed in Workout # 3, when children are expected to follow in their parent's footsteps without regard for their own interests, abilities, and passions, children don't feel they have a voice. Often, they don't feel as though they matter.

- **Pilates Pointer:** Introduce a variety of interests to your children. Allow them to pursue their passions. Guide and support them as they develop competence. As they continue to explore and produce, affirm their worth and acknowledge their contributions.

Stage Five (12 - 18 years): Role Confusion vs. Identity

For any parent or guardian who has been here, this is when parenting is put to the test! As difficult as it is for parents and guardians, this is an incredibly challenging time for teens. During this stage of development, teens area finding out who they are and what they are all about. Teens must be given the freedom to explore different paths and different roles within those paths. Developing a secure identity also requires teens learn to define themselves based on their internal sources of worth: abilities, interests, beliefs, values, etc. It is critical parents and guardians serve as effective mentors, providing opportunities and guiding them during this time of inner-personal evaluation and exploration. As teens pursue different avenues and paths, they must individuate from their parents or guardians. In other words, during this stage it is important teens begin to see themselves as unique, separate individuals (different from their parents and guardians) who are learning to make their own choices and accepting responsibility for them. As teens discover what is important to them and derive a purposeful path to follow, then a positive identify will take hold.

Parents and guardians want the best for their teens. They want them to be safe, successful, and well-adjusted. However, many times parents and guardians impose a predetermined path on their teens, or expect them to be someone they are not, or they hold onto the parental reigns too tightly. When teens are not given the freedom to individuate, they are less likely to develop their real or true identities. By not living out a path which is congruent with their interests, beliefs, and values, teens experience identity confusion.

- **Pilates Pointer:** Allow your teens the freedom to detach from parental control, to explore their interests, and to discover who they are and what is important to them. Encourage them to be true to themselves and to the passions they want to pursue, supporting them in the healthy paths they select.

In conclusion, in recent years research has supported how children are launching much later than previous generations. They are staying home longer and often returning home after time away. As we have discussed in "Pilates For Parenting", keep the communication channels open. Stay connected. Listen to your children, teens, and young adults. Really listen and seek to understand them. If you see they are struggling or are stuck, it is only natural for parents and guardians to want to fix everything for them or to take away their pain. It is never too late to address past injuries, injustices, or insecurities; however, sometimes it requires trusting your children, teens, and young adults to the expertise of a professional therapist or counselor. It is important they do their own healing work. As a seasoned Pilates Parent, love and accept them along the way.

About the Author

Holli Kenley is a California Licensed Marriage and Family Therapist and a California State Licensed Teacher. She holds a Master's Degree in Psychology with an emphasis in Marriage, Family, and Child Counseling. She has worked in a variety of settings: a women's shelter, a counseling center, and in private practice. Counseling with teens, adults, and couples, Holli's areas of specialized training and experience include sexual abuse and trauma, betrayal, codependency, cyber bullying, and screen addiction. After relocating to Southern California, Holli reopened her private practice in Rancho Mirage.

Holli Kenley is the author of eight recovery books including:

- *Breaking Through Betrayal: And Recovering The Peace Within, 2nd Edition*

- *Power Down & Parent Up: Cyber Bullying, Screen Dependence & Raising Tech-Healthy Children*

- Holli is also a contributing author and Wellness Editor for *Clear Life Magazine*.

Holli Kenley, M.A., MFT, also works in the field of psychology as an author, speaker, and workshop presenter. She has been a six time peer presenter at the California Association of Marriage and Family Therapists' Annual State Conferences and a featured or keynote speaker at college level clinical programs, state and national advocacy organizations, and educational institutions speaking on the topics of bullying, cyber bullying, betrayal, relapse, screen dependency, sexual abuse recovery, and the power of self-worth. Holli has been a guest on over 100 podcasts as well as on Arizona TV speaking on issues of wellness. Prior to and during her career as a therapist, Holli taught for thirty years in public education.

Holli lives in Southern California with her husband.

To contact Holli Kenley for your next workshop or presentation, visit www.hollikenley.com.

Bibliography

Abbate, E. (2019). 8 Things to know before you take pilates. *Self*, (January). https://www.self.com

Alter, A. (2017). *Irresistible: The rise of addictive technology and the business of keeping us hooked*. New York, NY: Penguin Press.

Bandura, A. (2015). *Moral disengagement: How people do harm and live with themselves*. New York, NY: Worth Publishers.

Bosker, B. (2016). Tristan Harris believes silicon valley is addicting us to our phones: And he's determined to make it stop. *The Atlantic*, (November),56-65.

Briere, J. & Scott, C. (2015). *Principles of trauma therapy: A guide to symptoms, evaluation, and treatment (DSM -5 update) 2nd edition*. Los Angeles, CA: Sage Publications.

David, L. "Erikson's Stages of Development," in *Learning Theories*, July 23, 2014, https://www.learning-theories.com/eriksons-stages-of-development.html

Dunckley, V, L. MD. (2015). *Reset your child's brain: A four-week plan to end meltdowns, raise grades and boost social skills by reversing the effects of electronic screen-time*. Novato, CA: New World Library.

Felt, L. J., & Robb, M.B., (2016). Technology addiction Concern, controversy, and finding balance. *Common Sense – Executive Summary*, (May), 3-13. Retrieved January, 2017.

Gold, G.D. (2018). *I will be complete: A memoir*. New York, NY: Random House, LLC (Alfred A. Knopf).

Grossman, D.., & DeGaetano. G. (2014). *Stop teaching our kids to kill: A call to action against tv, movie, and video game violence*. New York, NY: Harmony Books (Crown Publishing Group).

Heid, M. (2016). Devices mess with your brain…Is your smartphone affecting your mind? Yes – and you're probably suffering from phantom text syndrome, too. *Time – Special Edition*. 34-37.

Herzanek, J. (2016). *Why don't they just quit: Hope for families struggling with addiction*. Berthoud, CO: Changing Lives Foundation.

Kabali, H. K., Irigoyen, M.M., Nunez-Davis, R., et al (2015). Exposure and use of mobile media devices by young children. *American Academy of Pediatrics*, 136 (6). Retrieved January 2017.

Kardaras, N. (2016) *Glow Kids: How screen addiction is hijacking our kids – and how to break the trance. (*First ed.). New York, N.Y: St. Martin's Press.

Kenley, H. (2015). *Another way – a novel.* Ann Arbor: Loving Healing Press, Inc.

Kenley, H. (2016). *Breaking through betrayal: And recovering the peace within 2nd edition.* Ann Arbor: Loving Healing Press, Inc.

Kenley, H. (2018). *Daughters betrayed by their mothers: Moving from brokenness to wholeness.* Ann Arbor, MI: Loving Healing Press, Inc.

Kenley, H. (2013). *Mountain air: Relapsing and finding the way back... one breath at a time.* Ann Arbor: Loving Healing Press, Inc.

Kenley, H. (2017). *Power down and parent up: Cyber bullying, screen dependence, & raising tech-healthy children.* Ann Arbor, MI: Loving Healing Press, Inc.

Kenley, H. Healthy friendships: Part one: are mine easy? Part two: are mine equal? Part three: are mine enriching? Clear Life Magazine. https://clearlifemagazine.com/read/wellness/ 2018.

Kersting, T. (2016). *Disconnected: How to reconnect our digitally distracted kids.* USA: Thomas Kersting.

Koch, K. (2015). *Screens and teens: Connecting with our kids in a wireless world.* Chicago: Moody Press.

Nichols, M. P. (2014). *Family therapy: Concepts and methods.* Harlow: Pearson.

Rideout, V. (2017). *The Common Sense census: Media use by kids age zero to eight.* San Francisco, CA: Common Sense Media. Retrieved December 2017.

Salvador, M., & Vetere, A. (2012). *Families and family therapy.* London: Routledge.

Santrock, J. W. (2014). *A topical approach to life-span development.* Boston: McGraw-Hill.

Scheck, S. (2014) *The stages of psychosocial development according to Erik Erikson.* Norderstedt, Germany: GRIN Publishing.

Strasburger, V.C., & Hogan, M.J., 92013). *Children, adolescents, and the media* [Abstract]. American Academy of Pediatrics, 132 November), 958-961. Retrieved January 10, 2017.

Taughinbaugh, C. (2014). *Parents to PhDs: 28 interviews with parents who share heartache, wisdom, and healing through first-hand experiences.* (Kindle ed.). Amazon Digital Services.

Twenge, J. (2017). *iGen: Why today's super-connected kids are growing up less rebellious, more tolerant, less happy – and completely unprepared for adulthood* and what that means for the rest of us.* New York: ATRIA Books.

Index

Electronic Media Can Endanger As Well As Empower Your Kids

In this decade, our digital world has grown exponentially as has the degree of time both adults and children are spending on their screens. Not surprisingly, researchers are discovering a myriad of unhealthy behaviors associated with excessive screen time. In *Power Down & Parent Up*, Kenley expands on her groundbreaking book *Cyber Bullying No More*, giving parents/guardians effective strategies to integrate into their lives and their children's. How can we navigate a tech-driven world and raise tech-healthy children?

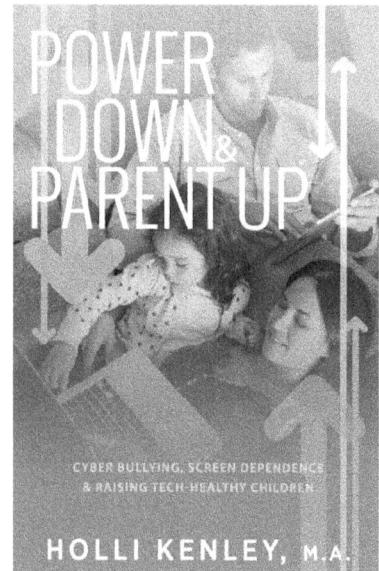

- Tackle cyber bullying head-on by implementing a concise "Parent Up" approach with proven strategies for *Protection, Intervention, and Prevention.*

- "Power Down" on screen dependence and become fully informed about its growing health concerns and consequences.

- Learn *Seven Proactive Practices* such as goal setting and creating a family plan to reduce screen time.

- Discover *Four Healthy Guidelines* to add to our parenting toolbox such as learning how to communicate about the false nature of cyber worth and cultivate our children's real worth.

"Rather imply that families can return to some idealistic less complicated time without Facebook, sexting, social networks, and Twitter, and whatever else comes along, Kenley's booklet will help parents mitigate possible harm to their children as they integrate this technology hopefully into healthy lives and relationships."
--Ronald Mah, M.A. LMFT, author of *Difficult Behavior in Early Childhood* and *The One Minute Temper Tantrum Solution*

"Holli addresses children's readiness for technology as well as rules, contracts and education for parents to consider for their children as they introduce or allow entry of new technology into their lives. Cyber bullying and victimization are concerns addressed as well as internet resources for parents, with tools for protection, interventions and prevention--a must for parents in our technological world."
--Lani Stoner, Marriage and Family Therapist

paperback * hardcover * eBook * audiobook

Learn more at www.HolliKenley.com

High school. Dating. Sex. 14 yr old Chloe Wheeler wonders - is she ready?

Finding it uncomfortable talking with her parents, Chloe turns to her best friend--Amanda Hill. Searching for guidance, they attend a nondenominational youth group where Pastor Rick Summers is facilitating a series of talks on sex entitled Another Way. At the first group meeting, Chloe meets football star Tyrell Fields. As they begin dating and Chloe's feelings intensify, she grabs hold of the lessons of *Another Way* and discovers...

- Her worth.
- Her voice.
- Her levels of readiness.
- Her power to make healthy decisions.

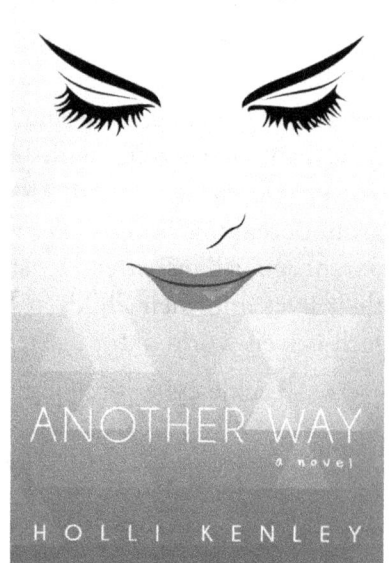

ANOTHER WAY
a novel

HOLLI KENLEY

"Holli Kenley beautifully shares in *Another Way* how young people can embrace confidence and self-empowerment as they find their way through the challenges of the teen years."

Cathy Taughinbaugh--Parent Coach, Helping Parents Find Peace

"*Another Way* is an indispensable book for teens and those who care about them...Holli Kenley has done it again with this practical, entertaining, and bold book."

Jill Osborne, Eds, LPC, RPT - Helping Families Reconnect

"*Another Way* introduces our young readers to a new way of thinking. Through self-discovery and self-empowerment, Chloe learns there truly is Another Way--a way to stand strong with honesty and personal integrity."

Judy Herzanek – Changing Lives Foundation

"*Another Way* is one of those great reads that is sure to find an audience with readers of all ages."

Cyrus Webb – Host of *Conversations Live*, Editor-in-Chief *Conversations Magazine*

paperback * hardcover * eBook

Learn more at www.HolliKenley.com

The daughters' stories touch upon the deepest and darkest of pains: knowing you have a mother... but you don't.

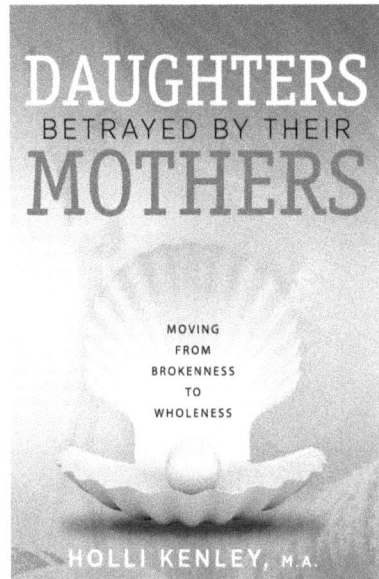

Daughters Betrayed By Their Mothers: Moving From Brokenness To Wholeness is an intimate exploration into the lives of daughters who were wounded by their mothers and who chose wellness over victimhood. Each daughter's unique story of recovery is a testament to the power of choice, perseverance and resilience. Readers are invited to journey alongside the daughters, grabbing hold of healing lifelines and moving from broken places to whole spaces within.

- Do you feel your mother did not "show up" for you in the ways you needed?

- Because of your mother's role in your life, do you feel like you were "not enough?"

- Do you wonder if it is possible to heal from the brokenness that comes from being wounded by your mother?

If you answered "yes" to any of these questions, the "Daughters" warmly welcome you.

"There are tears of both sorrow and joy in the beautiful, brave stories of harm and hope. Daughters Betrayed By Their Mothers changed my life."
--Charlotte Carson, Editorial Director, ClearLifeMagazine.com

"*Daughters Betrayed By Their Mothers* is heartrending and uplifting; dark and optimistic; painful and inspirational. A profound human document."
--Sam Vaknin, author of *Malignant Self-Love: Narcissism Revisited*

"Powerful, reflective, and reassuring to all who read it, Holli Kenley's *Daughters Betrayed By Their Mothers* reminds us that no matter what hurt we have experienced, the opportunity to heal and be whole is always possible."
--Cyrus Webb, media personality, author, and speaker

paperback * hardcover * eBook * audiobook

Learn more at www.HolliKenley.com